The Bicycle Effect

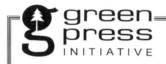

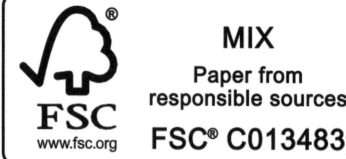

The Bicycle Effect
Cycling as Meditation

Juan Carlos Kreimer

FINDHORN PRESS

Bici Zen – Ciclismo urbano como meditación
© by Juan Carlos Kreimer, 2011, 2016
by Agreement with Guenter G. Rodewald (mercadodelibros.info)
English translation © Findhorn Press, 2016

Originally published by Editorial Planeta, Argentina, 2013.

ISBN 978-1-84409-708-1

A CIP record for this title is available from the British Library.

Translation by Nick Inman
Edited by Nicky Leach
Illustrations by Simona Golinelli,
with kind permission of Rayuela Edizioni, Italy
Front cover design by Richard Crookes
Interior design by Thierry Bogliolo
Printed and bound in the USA

Published by
Findhorn Press
117-121 High Street,
Forres IV36 1AB,
Scotland, UK
t +44 (0)1309 690582
f +44 (0)131 777 2711
e info@findhornpress.com
www.findhornpress.com

Contents

Foreword   *by Joan Garriga Bacardi*   7
Introduction   A Beautiful Feeling of Nothing   17

Part I: A Long Way to Cycle
        The Phenomenon, the Opportunity   23
1. The Urban Cyclist   25

Part II: I Celebrate Your Inner Bike
        Doing It, Enjoying It   63
2. Riding   65
3. Wake Up, Energy!   111
4. Man – Bike – Way   123

Part III: Rules of Experience
        Care, Meaning   141
5. Right Riding   143
6. Look Out   155
7. Keep It Impeccable   161

Epilogue 1:   My Seven Bikes   170
Epilogue 2:   Secular Zen   182
Bibliography   189
Acknowledgements   191
About the Author   192

*"A man is rich in proportion
to the number of things he can afford to let alone."*
— *H. D. Thoreau*

*"Tension is who you think you should be.
Relaxation is who you are."*
—*Zen Saying*

Foreword

When I ride a bike, I ride a bike

Each November, when I pass through Buenos Aires, it has become a sort of ritual for me to meet Juan Carlos Kreimer in a bar in the Plaza Serrano, in the lively neighbourhood of Palermo. He normally arrives on his bicycle, wearing a blue cap, and with the bottom of his right trouser leg held by a clip, to keep it clear of the oil and grease of the chain.

There is no doubt that Juan Carlos has had a long and special relationship with his bike. He touches it with a sense of affection and familiarity that makes me think of those couples who, despite the passing of the years, are still interested in each other; who desire and respect each other; and experience a lovely, natural way of co-operating, as if they were not two people but one. It would be an exaggeration to say that Juan Carlos and his bike are one, but I wouldn't want to say that they are two. There is something special between them.

I have known Juan Carlos for around 25 years, and I have seen how he gives his passion and energy to everything that moves him, and that he loves. So I am not surprised at all that he has decided to write a book about cycling and Zen, as he is certainly a seeker after consciousness who has explored the ins and outs of many therapeutic and spiritual techniques, combining both things, and he has an obvious talent for integrating knowledge from different sources.

I met him when he was editing the magazine *Uno Mismo*. In it, he published one of my first articles, which greatly reassured me, because its title referred to the therapist as "priest" and "prostitute", words not usually used in the terrain of psychotherapy. I am still grateful for that because, to my surprise and incredulity, I noticed that afterwards my colleagues paid more attention to me than before—something new for me, given that I hadn't identified myself much with the majority of texts that I had written.

Then he came to Barcelona, to the Gestalt Institute, to lead a workshop entitled Rebecoming Men, which is the title of one of his books. The subject of "being men" occupied his interest and attention for several years. I have always thought that he is motivated by a reliable inner radar that makes him interested in a variety of subjects to do with thoughts and actions that help and transform us.

Over the years, a trusting friendship has grown up between us. It is one of those friendships that finds its strength and beauty in distance and, probably because of this, is all the more valuable and generous—one of those much appreciated brotherly connections in the journey of life for which I am truly grateful. Montaigne was so right when he remarked: "A life without friends is like life on a desert island. True friendship multiplies the good in life and divides its evils. It is the only remedy against ill fortune, and a relief for the soul."

We greet each other, sit in a cafe, talk for a while about the essentials of life, projects, interests, loves, comings and goings, troubles, and various stages of the journey. We listen to each other, and we talk about practical ways that we can make life easier, such as, above all, to know that there is someone there. Then we say goodbye until the next time we meet, without knowing how or when that will be. And I see him leave with his blue cap, his smile, his air of happiness, and his bike. Or I accompany him for some blocks in whichever direction he is going—the last time he took me to visit the centre near Plaza Serrano, where he helps others to write and to know themselves through writing, another of his specialties.

Searching my bad memory, I cannot remember whether it was during one of these talks in a cafe, or via email, that he asked me to write a foreword to his book in which I could say whatever I wanted. I accepted enthusiastically—out of friendship, brotherhood, and, above all, because I have faith. Having faith means a lot to me. It means trusting that whatever a person does, he does it from a good place. The same thing happens to me with therapists. I do not need to see them work; I just need to know whether I have faith in them or not. What does it depend on? It seems to be something very unscientific, such as perceiving them to be benevolent or having the spontaneous desire to make others feel good about themselves. The rest—the work they do—is an extension of this, or an addition to it.

What follows are some reflections about the impact this book has had on me, and about the essence that remains with me.

After finishing reading *The Bicycle Effect*, I am left wondering whether it offers words to live by in the world or literature for what we could call the "transcendent self". Does it deal with stimuli related to the affairs of everyday life, or is it about spiritual matters?

The response on one level is: both. It combines an invitation to enjoy life on two wheels—this mystery of simply being alive which, if we are fortunate, we experience as simply a "free" opportunity—along with a lot of practical advice on the art of riding a bike and nutrients and poetry to feed the spirit provided by the immense wisdom of Zen. It suggests that we drop our fixations and, instead, nurture a sense of attention, emptiness, non-doing, mindfulness, full presence, and hygiene of thought, all of which can induce greater compassion, which in turn leads to greater happiness, even though this is a spontaneous benefit that we didn't set out to seek.

There is no doubt that compassion is crucial. We should remember that Buddhism evolved from small

plained in the book) that is used more and more each day. New recruits are attracted by what it represents: think independently, simplify things, slow down, see, feel, keep in contact with yourself and with life. It is as if it embodies an emblematic principle that sums up a set of values and sensations, including being in harmony with nature, health, care, respect, simplicity, human rhythm, humanity, enjoyment, childhood and curiosity, balance, self-reliance, environmental awareness, and so forth. It barely pollutes. It doesn't make you stupid. It doesn't release toxic gases. And in its care and repair, you can make yourself almost self-sufficient because its mechanics are simple and do not depend on big business or on highly specialized professionals. Skilled bicycle sale and repair shops often thrive as small businesses and retain a flavour of the handmade, family-run, and customer-friendly.

Taking the analogy of bicycling being non-polluting and "pure" further: When you ride a bike, and you are swept up in the flow of what you are doing, or even feel one with the bike and the environment and with what is happening in each moment, the mind is released from its fog and its toxins and, so to speak, is purified: it becomes empty like the clear blue sky, and consequently peaceful. The cyclist smiles. All the mental constructions and residues that make up your model of the world—views, analyses, categories, and so on—are dissolved, or at least placed on hold. Paradoxically, the model or map of the world that we create separates us from it. It is important, therefore, to let go of it and purify yourself.

Mark 8:35, in the New Testament, tells us that to die to the world is to attain eternal life: "For whosoever will save his life shall lose it; but whosoever shall lose his life for my sake and the gospel's, the same shall save it." It is beautiful—the idea that through riding a bike, which is in motion, you can experience a stationary and eternal present, empty yourself out, even as the future approaches us and absorbs us with its capricious forms.

As I have said, this book contains nutrients and poetry for the spirit. Reading it led me to reread the poem *Faith in Mind* (*Shin Jin Mei* in Japanese) by the master Sosan, third Zen patriarch. Once again, I was struck by this wonderful and cryptic poem: "Make the least distinction and heaven and earth are separated infinitely."

This is what he says about purification. The thing that creates singularities, distinctions, or evaluations is thought, by taking you away from the contemplative mode and slicing up reality (not to say dismembering it) with its conceptual axe. In this way, heaven and earth, light and darkness, up and down, form and emptiness cease to be one and the same; we enter duality—dichotomy and dialectic. The "I" establishes itself and builds its own prison. Zen is method and goal at the same time. It is not a means to an end, but a simultaneous means and an end. It offers the potential to break the walls of our personal prison.

As an aside, this evocative book led me back into my personal past. On cold and boring evenings in Pamplona, during periods of leave from the stupid barracks where I did my stupid military service, I read Suzuki Roshi. I am sure that I did not understand much, but I didn't care, because simply reading it gave me a sensation of feeling more alive, more in myself, or something like that; and it acted as an antidote to the time-wasting and meaninglessness of the military. Today, I think that, without being fully aware of it, I was motivated by this desire for transcendence and wisdom that I believe lives and beats in all of us.

Coming back to bicycles, memories of my rural childhood have flooded back while reading this book. I was part of a large family, and I have a clear memory (as well as the emotions attached) of the one-of-a-kind children's bike at my grandparents' farmhouse, which was used by a huge number of cousins, all eager to ride 300 metres of glory, before passing it on with regret, unwillingness, and envy to the next child. With so many brothers and cousins, we had to learn generosity, respect, and sharing. But the yearning and pleasure associated with riding that bike were indescribable, pedalling along the track, flanked by almond trees and reeds, until you reached the point where for safety reasons you had to turn back in order to avoid the railway line that ran through the small village.

I was also taken back to my grandfather's enormous, old, yellowish-orange bike. If we saw his parked bike while he was drinking coffee and playing cards in the bar beside the park, we would run to ask if we could take turns riding it. We had to put our right legs inside the frame to climb onto the saddle and then we could start pedalling. Later, I felt the enormous teenage pleasure of pedalling with groups of friends around the roads that surround the fields.

I realize now that I did not have my own bicycle until I was a grown-up. I bought my first one in Barcelona when I was 20 years old. I confess that after using it a little in the city, I was scared and became convinced that my life was in imminent danger. Fortunately, times have changed, and today there are increasing numbers of bike lanes and people adding themselves to the ranks of urban cycling, inspired by the stress reduction and health benefits that bicycle-friendly cities promote.

I am grateful to Juan Carlos for his words, which have brought back fond memories that were deeply buried under layers of duty and responsibility. He has also reminded me of the wise words of Galeano: "Live only to live, just as the bird sings without knowing that it is singing or as the child plays without knowing that it is playing". Another confession: after reading the book I have gone back to riding a bike for pleasure.

I will conclude by saying that this is an inspired and fascinating book, humanist and countercultural, intellectual and experiential, rigorous and loving, intelligent and accessible, earthly and spiritual. And above all, a book of Zen, whose simplest, most sophisticated, and least intelligible maxim (as the book reminds us) is, "When I eat, I eat. When I sleep, I sleep." To which I would add, "When I ride a bike, I ride a bike."

Joan Garriga Bacardi,

August 2015, Port de la Selva

Humanistic psychologist
Founder of Institut Gestalt of Barcelona;
Expert in Family Constellation work;
Author of *Vivir en el Alma*
and *El buen amor en la pareja*

Introduction

A Beautiful Feeling of Nothing

If you have ever got on your bike and started pedalling and felt that your actions were independent of your will, and that everything you were thinking about was put on pause, I don't need to explain what I mean. Zen calls this being fully present.

It is the end of 1982, and I am 38 years old. One day, at noon, I notice that my bike is steering itself. Later, I am sitting on the bay, which is today occupied by the Memorial Garden, facing the Rio de la Plata. With me is Daniel Coifman, a psychotherapist friend who has spent a couple of seasons at the Esalen Institute of Big Sur, travelled several times to India and, to put it briefly, gone exploring the mysteries of consciousness. Our bicycles are leaning against each other.

I tell him that I can remember all the places that we have been: the Planetarium, the level crossing, near the airport, the crossroads near the Fishermen's Club. Also, the wind on my face, the water splashing the railings, the smell of food at the restaurants when you made a detour to avoid the two elderly people who were drinking maté... However, I do not remember the thoughts that I had. I was distracted. I didn't know where I was. I only knew in that moment that "I am here".

Daniel jumps up. "No, you were not distracted," he says. "You were abstracted, but you were not absent. And believe it or not, it is exactly the opposite."

Thirty years have passed since that beautiful feeling of nothing and that conversation next to the river. Five notebooks of 160 pages each, almost broken from so much putting in and taking out of my pocket, have been filled with hundreds of words and disconnected phrases, prayers, and unfinished paragraphs, copied or underlined quotations. From time to time, I copy them into a long file on my computer and open it at any page:

- "The traveller is the engine."
- "There are risks, not ghosts."
- "Get involved without being involved."

The connections between bike and Zen come by themselves, no matter which areas of life they refer to. I don't look for them; they follow me.

Meditation does not mean sitting cross-legged, palms upwards, trying to reach another mental state; to sit is that state. In the same way, sitting with your legs hanging down, moving to the rhythm of the pedals, and with your hands on the handlebars, is in itself the mental state of the bike.

The two practices are forms of "mental digestion", because they purify us inside. They may seem to entail a passive silence, but it is not so, because the mind empties itself and naturally enters a subtle state of attention.

The information that the cyclist communicates to the bike, and that the bike returns to him, creates a dialogue similar to the one we have with our bodies, whose parts anticipate the messages of the mind and seem to move with autonomy.

A hand runs along the edge of a table and recognizes where it ends. A leg in the air and a movement of the foot are capable of receiving a football and directing it towards the free angle of the goal—all this in less than a second, as if no one asks the mind what to do, and the mind doesn't take a decision.

The mind performs a double function: it is there taking care of things and also sending the required assistance (information). It is engaged in a choreography that transcends all vocabulary.

When connected to the senses, the bike as an object becomes an extension of your body, as if it were another limb. It manages to convey its state—what it needs in any moment—and interprets the impulses it receives from the brain of the rider through the points of contact. We establish such a dialogue almost as soon as we learn to ride. It becomes instinctive, and we do not realize it.

In Zen, riding *is* that dialogue.

In the same way, when the body and mind are combined—from now on, we will say aligned—the flow of energy or vital *élan* encounters fewer obstructions. It naturally comes and goes within the rider, and the bike and the contact points between the two act as interfaces.

When we meditate, the different bodies that we are composed of (physical, emotional, mental, and others less perceptible, such as subtle body energies) are aligned. This cancels out the interference of the mind and allows the consciousness to establish a nonverbal contact with our deepest essence. Sometimes we attain peaks not reached by any thought, and it seems to us that we are simultaneously present and not present. There is no difference between the observed and the fact that it is we who are observing. We can stay there or go farther and return when we want.

Although wanting to reach that state on a bike can be dangerous, to tune into meditation is to take advantage of every opportunity to fully integrate the continuum of man-bike-way (way, here, including the environment).

This perspective makes greater sense now that cycling has become a widespread practice, part of daily life and increasingly accepted. Many people are discovering that travelling by bike does more than serve their physical needs; it is also a method of internal alignment.

The mechanic who fixes my car is also a cyclist and he says, "When I need alignment and balancing, I go out on that old banger," and he points to a black bike leaning against the wall at the back of his garage.

Part I

A Long Way to Cycle

The Phenomenon, the Opportunity

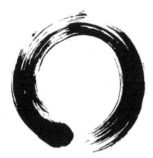

1

The Urban Cyclist

Bikes have become part of everyday life.
The majority are used more for recreation
than as a means of transport.
Almost all the cities of the world have modified
their street layouts to encourage and protect cyclists.
The bicycle goes beyond the spaces
allocated to it by the authorities;
it transcends popularity and fashion;
and its use has become contagious.
What appears to be a form is a content.
Whichever way it is used, it creates habit.

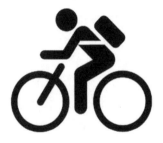

Ancestors of the Bike

From the Neolithic period, when it was discovered that a round shape was able to roll, there was no one stopping the movement. Perhaps man already knew—as we know these things that we do not know that we know—that the wheel hid a greater purpose, another fruit of Creation destined to be tested.

Apparently, man could now give a boost to his yearning to go faster than his feet would carry him, and much farther.

The famous human proportion perfectly fitting in the squared circle was turned in profile and, in 1490, enabled Leonardo Da Vinci to design a prototype bicycle down to its exact anatomy and dynamic. With the same eye that wanted to see the man move through the air like a bird, Leonardo imagined a system of auto-propulsion that would enable a man to fly 15 centimetres (6 inches) from the ground. The Carrousell, a model not very different from the classic bike of the 20th century, includes steering directly linked to the handlebar, pedals at the base of the frame, and a chain drive! It fits and supports the human body perfectly, which is placed in a ideal position to hold the bike, drive it forward, and become one with it.

Around 1880, when the Englishman John Kemp Starley started to produce his so-called "safety bicycles", featuring a chain of articulated links between the pedal and the back wheel, Da Vinci must have been shouting from the grave, "At last, boys!"

The difference in size between the highest number of teeth of the chain wheel in relation with those on the gear sprockets enabled improvements: for each turn of the pedals, it revolved more times and the wheel turned faster.

The idea of transmission and multiplication was irreplaceable, but having the gear of the rear wheel fixed to the axle was not ideal. The advantage: it allowed the bike to get to speed in just a few metres and to brake using the legs without lowering the feet to the ground. Against: it was impossible to stop pedalling. When the rider stopped applying force through his legs, the pedals and the chain were kept moving by the momentum of the rear wheel. Very shortly afterwards, another Englishman invented the freewheel, a sort of clutch that allowed the rider to disconnect the legs from the traction. All bikes today, whether with or without gears, use fundamentally the same system.

Bicycles began to be mass-produced on both sides of the Atlantic, and colonies adopted them as a sign of progress. Cycling ceased to be a practice reserved for elite males, and the bike became a vehicle of transport.

During the 20th century, the bike conformed to the Biblical premise of "increase and multiply"—notionally, at least. But it did so with a minimum of Darwinism, because the principle of a diamond-shaped frame has barely evolved since then. Bikes have been given a greater or lesser amount of metal tubes, and these have been made more upright or more curved. Bicycle designs also vary, according to what is on show or not. In essence, however, the bike is always based on the same triangle built around saddle, pedals, and handlebar to support the same three points of contact: buttocks, feet, and hands. With all its variants, the bike still responds to the human profile taken as a basis by Leonardo Da Vinci.

Objects of Cult

"He handled the bike with kid gloves, you might say.
He would always see to it that neither front
nor back wheel wobbled. Often he would do
a job for me without pay, because, as he put it,
he never saw a man so in love with his bike as I was."
—*Henry Miller,* My Bike and Other Friends

Can some objects such as the bicycle be alive? Especially machines without an engine that complement human functions, such as old lawn mowers or pedal-operated sewing machines?

As with musical instruments, bikes do not have an energy that we can see, only that which passes through their mechanisms—that comes from our feet or hands (the push we give them) or from a slope. They stream-line physical laws such as gravity, balance, inertia, the centrifugal force. They multiply forces, process infor-mation, combine different forces, and adapt them-selves to different situations. They carry us—they put up with our excess weight, our skills, our vices, our whims. They lead us. They understand us...

And on more subtle planes, they also have some-thing, some of *that*, an abstract quality that humans have never been able to name. I am referring to *that which is beyond us*.

To want to determine whether their spirit is born of their essence or their function is the same as pretend-ing that the observer can be independent of what he observes or the mind separated from the I. It is innate, since it was there from its inception.

Every bike has a personality and is the subject of a private cult. Each person builds a relationship with his bike, whatever it is like, in the same way as with a favourite pair of shoes or T-shirt, even though there are thousands of similar objects in existence. A model of the same brand does not have the same effect. Each person establishes his own relationship.

It is a relationship in the body. As in all body-to-body interactions, there are factors that go beyond the mind. Whoever gets on a bike perceives how it receives him, how it supports his weight, what it requires, how it responds to his stimuli. Not all models cause the same feeling of completeness. Once the empathy is established, there comes feedback and then the rider can relax. It is an alchemy that is a surrender or a forgetting of the self. It provides release and other feelings similar to those that occur during sexual intercourse.

Riding a bike does not oblige you to rationalize each movement; the dynamic of it makes you do what is appropriate. First I go forward, then I think about it. As with playing a musical instrument, habits operate at a subconscious level. When the performer reaches a certain degree of rapport, he is immersed in the euphoria of the execution and cannot pause to reflect how or what he is doing. He gives himself to the music, as the cyclist gives himself to the ride.

On reading the last paragraph, Nicholas Muszkat writes in the margin: "When I was 32 years old (two years ago), I went with my father to the bicycle shop we used in my childhood. Miguelito, the owner, showed me a bike hanging up. It was almost a wreck. 'You had one like this, just the same,' he said. It was a 20" Aurorita folding bicycle. All the parts were made in Argentina, even the brakes. Of course, I bought it and restored it. I now get the same pleasure from bikes as I did when I first learned to ride one."

For anyone who loved bikes as a child, the bike never dies and no bicycle dies completely. It may be dismembered and the parts thrown away, but there will always be someone who rescues a rusty frame before it goes on the recycling truck and rebuilds it with odd pieces or discarded parts taken from other bikes. It is rare that the tubes end up being scrapped; they always reincarnate and come back to relive the connection between the cyclist and the bike.

The anthropologist Marc Augé considers it a bond of love and, literally, of recognition, which time does not destroy, but rather strengthens through memories and nostalgia, even if life has separated the bike from its owner.

It is a metaphor of an existence based on a utopian balance between man and nature; a longing for a golden age not defiled by commercialism; a freedom that can be symbolically recovered. The bike conjures up many associations...

The Imperceptible

At the end of the eighties, when almost all bicycle manufacturers, American and European, began to offer models with integrated gear changing systems, very few people realized that this was something more than a technological innovation. "They respond in a way by understanding, and putting into practice, the act of riding a bike, including reading conscious automatic movements, however small they may be," Nicolas Muszkat explains to me. He is the man who restored his childhood bike and who is now the Latin American manager for Shimano, the brand responsible for the majority of gears operating throughout the world. He points out that they are not added to the bike just so that the cyclist can apply more or less force; their purpose is for the rider to be able to do this without distracting his attention. They become a part of his body, the same as the air he breathes, without realizing it.

The imperceptible, as a concept implicit in the gear changer, points directly to the way that the reaction of the cyclist is applied with the least possible intervention of his thinking. It happens at the same moment as the sensory data reaches his mind, and it is separate from the act of will to decide to change gear. The rider does not even realize what he is doing, just as when he squeezes the brakes without thinking in response to an alert. In Japanese martial arts terms, when such a close union between the instrument and its function is achieved, the energy could be said to "activate itself".

Is it a coincidence that the factories from which this impressive engineering derives, and the company headquarters, are in Sakai, a city in the province of Osaka, where the four elements characteristic of the tea ceremony—harmony, reverence, purity, calm—form a counterpoint to the former steelworks that were used to make weapons?

Is it a coincidence that the founder of this company, Shozaburo Shimano, a man who knew the secrets of the cold-formed steel like the back of his own hand, alternated his work with fishing? He liked to do so alone, so that he could spend hours with the line just held between the thumb and forefinger, allowing his mind to be filled with nature...

Does any of this relate to the Zen spirit of cycling? I wonder.

Now that the bike has ceased to be a vehicle for romantics—and for fanatics—and has became an intelligent choice of transport, it provides the best bet for the sustainability of urban travel in the 21st century, and also offers the possibility of a healthy lifestyle. Cycling is a philosophy that can be put into practice. The bike survives as the last great invention of the mechanical age, whatever the innovations that are added to it: hinges so that it can be folded, electric motors with rechargeable batteries, frame designs without angles, new transporter models with the front wheel located a metre in front of the handlebar, and so on.

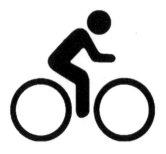

Awareness of the Road Network

No road network, no cyclists.

The cycling boom is opening up new challenges. Greater use of bikes and the creation of lanes for cyclists' safety need to be accompanied by the education of the cyclist. The notion of coexistence has to get inside the head that wears the helmet. In experiments, participants have been put into the role of drivers or pedestrians, so that they can learn to talk to each other. By understanding why other road users behave the way they do and how they see cyclists—and by listening without judgement to what they would say themselves if they could swap roles—it becomes clear that road users should be seen as complementing each other, rather than being in competition.

Without meaning to, these measures are an application of how Zen conceives of compassion: a way of understanding one another; whether we get about on foot or by bike, bus or 4x4 van, we are part of the same essence, and we are equally vulnerable. When a car runs over a bike, both are affected.

Seen in this way, the concrete traffic spacers that are taking over streets and avenues cease to be part of a policy to facilitate viability and provide security. They make those who go this way or that feel closer, more united. They are parts of the same network: the flow.

Compassion: Buddhas and bodhisattvas don't see compassion as feeling sorry for someone else; they agree that it is a feeling close to sympathy, that applies to both friends and enemies. If it is to be exercised with freedom, and lead to empathy and understanding and make energy circulate, it requires the wisdom that naturally emerges when we put aside ego and go beyond its limits.

Compassion operates as a network. One person does not give it while another receives it; both are channels for its energy.

It grows in the measure that it is practised.

The Inexplicable

*"The intrepid attitude of a hero
and the loving heart of a child."*
— Sôyen Shaku

Parents of adolescents in the city try as far as they can to deter them. They say, "Your body is your vehicle; it may be the other person's fault, but you will always bear the brunt. I know that you are careful... but the risk is other people." These are common phrases that have some truth to them. In the past and the present. The least touch from a car, and you lose your balance. When you are young, you graze your knees; when you are older, you may break some bone. Carelessness can be fatal.

But... how is it possible to live without using the bike? What can I replace it with? Sports are another thing.

"I'm not forbidding you, but don't say you weren't warned. When you take your bike I am worried..." As you ride, the backpack full of warnings is transformed into risk awareness. More than hearing a voice that paralyzes you or says, "Take care with this, watch out for that," you develop an intermittent state of alertness and attention.

You know where you are going and you learn to see without having to look. You understand the movements of the cars, and you make sure yours are predictable.

There is, in spite of everything, a heroic spirit in the urban cyclist. He is a David who risks his life going among Goliaths. Cars that come up behind and pass without paying attention; cars that overtake you without looking at who is moving alongside; parked cars that pull out a little to see if it is clear to drive away.

"Isn't it dangerous?" I am asked by a client who sees my helmet hanging off my backpack. He says it admiringly and warily, while thinking, *Why on earth does my editorial adviser travel by bike when he could get around in some other way.*

"Yes," I answer, while scenarios of accident and death parade through my mind, "but I am careful." As I say it, I am aware that I have to navigate between cars, motorcycles, buses, and lorries that go twice or three times my speed and weave in and out without the least consideration, and that only a touch from any one of them could knock me off. Nevertheless, there is a reason I cycle, which is difficult if not impossible to transmit.

"Don't you think there is something childish about continuing to do it?" Two streets from his offices, they have laid a two-lane bicycle track used by several men of our age. However, for him, as for the six out of every seven people that have not used a bike, so many bikes criss-crossing the city speaks of a need for independent transport. And, for anyone who wants to hear, it is also saying that each of us must construct his own happiness, individually, within a social system that contradicts even its own paradigms. There is no more time to dream of a utopia some day... You have to do it yourself by carrying out small daily acts, even if they are isolated—like having a vegetable patch at the bottom of the garden or separating the organic from the inorganic waste, or not leaving water running while we do the dishes. In these actions, we find an attitude that, little by little, permeates our lives.

I could also explain that there are at least two Juan Carloses who ride a bike: the child who once liked to feel the wind on his skin while he imagined flying, and a man with his feet on the ground that has already learnt some lessons. The joy in living of the three-year-old child who broke two milk teeth because he didn't know how to stop in time is still alive, even if it has had to contend with thousands of adaptations to life (and porcelain crowns). And this joy needs to come out.

My wife needs to go out on her bike to be out of doors. I am always far away—farther than far, said Federico Peralta Ramos, formulator of Gánica philosophy—while Sarita is riding her bike to the square. The word *Gánica* comes from *tener ganas*, to have desire. When you do what you really want, you may say you are *gánico*.

They are called "meta-needs". After meeting our primary security needs to eat, to have a roof over our heads, to feel loved, and to establish a tolerable level of self-esteem, the desire to live a full life brings to the surface needs that have been suppressed by the passage of time. Middle-aged people who have covered their basic needs often resort to pharmaceuticals to make them feel emotionally stable, secure, fulfilled, and satisfied—and to get them back to sleep when they wake at night.

The pills numb those feelings that come in abstract form or induce an indefinable feeling of emptiness. They make you think you are better. And yet, the mosquito continues to buzz.

Attaining freedom does not imply letting yourself go. It means making decisions: daring to leave behind the habits you are used to, which reappear automatically, because it is easier not to think about how much they influence you, because you are scared of trying something new, because you don't want to upset the conditioning that governs normality. It means allowing yourself to experiment, like a child, and to recognize your desires...

For many people, bicycling in the city elicits a fear that goes beyond all physical risk. It confronts them with a lifestyle that, little by little, they have been closing the doors on. It now comes under the category of activities that they are not allowed to do, or even to consider doing.

Others cannot deny its enchantment. After a few turns of the pedals, even if they are not aware of it, they start to experience moments of not thinking and of enjoyment, among other moments in which the mind dominates any kind of emotion. It awakens in them a memory of forgotten sensations in the body.

The feeling is incommunicable.

Working Up a Sweat

"To own a bike today is more chic
than owning a car:
it means that you live in the centre,
that you have free time. [...]
Our tastes are linked to a need
to differentiate ourselves from ordinary people."
—*Christian Boltanski*

It is true that my shirt is creased and hanging outside my trousers, that my hair is going every which way, that I have specks of grime between my fingers and at the corner of the eyes, and that I am wearing a certain expression of euphoria. Pedalling 10–15 kilometres (6–10 miles) an hour along 50 streets makes anyone scruffy.

My colleague is impeccable in his tweed jacket. He greets me with, "When you get rid of that Sunday smugness you arrived with, we can get started."

"Don't you see?" I ask, pretending to be surprised.

"I am more focussed than ever... What's more, on the way, I saw very clearly the places where we might get stuck."

I take my Mac laptop out of the backpack and place it on his desk. As I open it, I repeat to myself: "When I eat, I eat, and when I sleep, I sleep..." He begins to read aloud. I listen, with my eyes on my screen. Little by little, I'm forgetting how uncomfortable he makes me feel.

In that moment, I do not recognize the ghosts that I summon. I do not want him to accept my preferences. I just want him not to question them and to understand that I do not want to convince him of anything. He is he, I am I, and I have arrived on my bicycle to our weekly meeting. It doesn't mean that he has to do the same.

Almost three hours later, I return along the same cycle lane, going the other way. It is mid-afternoon, and many people are leaving work, equal numbers of men and women. Many of them seem to be going to some course. In front of me are two men with their briefcases strapped across their jackets like bandoliers. There is also a young mother with a girl in the rear seat and a lunchbox in the basket.

Why can some people do it? Why do they permit themselves to take the opportunity (express it how you want) and others don't?

The most common explanation is to refer to a concept of quality of life that is imposed from the outside. Advertising and the media feed the idea that a higher living standard is associated with having the best car, living in the most exclusive district, installing a big TV in your bedroom, having a mobile phone with more options, going to this or that exclusive tourist destination...

Advertisers and the media need to shower us with this type of message, because that is their reason for existence. If they put a bicycle at the bottom of an advertisement for clothing or devote a double page to the rise in popularity of cycling, it is because they know that it is identified with an emerging spirit of youth, with freedom, with environmentalism, with something vital, with quality of life, with a return to simplicity... and they seek to own it, as they do with any element or attitude that draws people to it. They do not include the bike for the love of using it, or because it stands for other changes of habits. In its widespread practice, they see future business.

In reality, the issue is more complex, because those who create the messages are no longer just the media, television no longer creates trends, and potential cyclists do not follow opinion leaders. No matter how many cool hunters the agencies hire, and no matter how many of the best creative people in the world turn up for brainstorming sessions to find ways to foster the mass acceptance of cycling, the number of bikes grows because of the behaviour of a small number of activists. By people who try it. One by one.

A picture (photo or drawing) of a house shows what it is. If you add one or two bicycles leaning, say, against a tree or a wall, the image indicates that there are people inside. Life.

As a symbol, the bike also reawakens the spirit of early childhood (between three and five years old) when the form is the content. The adult who sees the image of a bicycle, even though he is not a cyclist, allows himself a fleeting dream and nurtures a latent wish. It has some of the fantasy of flying.

In this subliminal corner of the imagination, never suppressed or acted on completely, any element of progress (and a culture built in accordance with this) is a trap. Americans express their inability to get out of the system with the word "bootstrap": pulling yourself up by the loops at the back of the boots. However much we try to escape from the consumerist behaviours that are imposed on us by techno-industrial Darwinism, the system always tempts us with objects and services that have become "artificial" needs. A very recent example: to be popular on Facebook.

The relatively new concept of "downsizing", which is the opposite of blind growth, is equivalent to that of "shedding", so essential to Zen. And the bike seems to be the best symbol for this.

The father is now short of breath. It hurts around his waist when he runs at the pace of the bike he has bought for his son. "Don't let go," shouts the child, when he feels the fatherly hand no longer on the saddle. In any case, he continues pedalling. Shortly before reaching the corner, he brakes, steers the bike in a new direction, and gets going again. His dad waves at him with the same hand that he was holding him with a moment ago. Suddenly, he can ride by himself. And he feels something new: freedom?

When we dream that we are riding a bicycle, there are three ways to understand the message. It can indicate making a personal effort beyond any other energy involved; it can speak to the notion of balance and the need for it to remain in motion; finally, it confirms that the journey is individual. The interpretations are superimposed; they may fork and intersect, but what is common to them all is the bike as a symbol of evolution in action.

In some dreams, its presence could be understood as depicting loneliness (psychological or real); or an excess of introversion or egocentricity; or a tendency to individualism that threatens to prevent the social integration of the cyclist. Although there may be something of this, the bike always corresponds to a normal need for autonomy. And it turns the wheel of Dharma: truths to be understood as expressions of reality as they happen, beyond personal expectations and preferences.

"I WILL CALL IT THE GROUND, EVERYTHING BELOW MY GAZE... AND HEAVEN EVERYTHING ABOVE." I saw this bumper sticker on the handlebars of a bike parked in front of a market for organic produce.

"What I save in train tickets, taxis, and fuel every month makes a difference," says a middle-aged man, while waiting for a green light. By his appearance and the toolbox he is carrying on the luggage rack, he may well be an electrician or handyman. He is riding a road bike that is more worn than mine. He finishes speaking while standing on the right pedal. An instant after, he becomes another cyclist seen from behind.

All motor vehicles connote urgency. Clock time dominates personal time. External time—from now or within half an hour, as quoted, and a scheduled return time. Time, common to all, in which we enter and exit in our own time. My colleague, the writer Juan Carlos Martelli, called the time that comes from your inner self rather than from outside, "time outside timetables".

Each person needs 15 square metres (160 square feet) and a ton and a half of resources (metals, plastics, fuels). The metropolis spends fortunes in infrastructure so that they can move around and be parked. At certain times of the day, they spend more time waiting than advancing. Even when they are not being used, they are expensive to maintain, and they depreciate. This is what they call comfort, the inhabitants of the first decades of the 21st century.

The cyclist is not a pedestrian with wheels, or a pedestrian who wants to go faster. Both are "blood-propelled", but in different ways. The person who travels by bike obtains a different kind of peace of mind to the one who travels on foot.

Twenty, 30, 40 streets still seem to me to be many streets. I can walk them, and with pleasure. From time to time I walk them with my wife, but I must (or she must) make me; I do not feel like going by myself.

When I get stuck with my writing, I'll use any excuse to go out for a walk. The mind adjusts to the walk with rhythmic breathing and allows me distance on the text I am working on. More than to oxygen, I attribute this to the "strainer effect": each step shakes up what has become stuck because of its consistency. I leave my house whistling an old song or repeating something that I believed I had forgotten, as if it were a mantra, and suddenly I begin to see how to untie the knot.

The emptiness that is created when I go out on my bike does not enable me to observe what I am doing from another point of view. It is a state of openness that looks forwards to new possibilities. The usual thoughts depart. My mind is freed from its conditioning, and it flowers with thoughts that only seconds before had been hidden at the back of my head.

The bicycle is a lonely pleasure, because almost no one talks while they ride. The thoughts come and go, and they are interspersed with the things that you see. It is rare to see a cyclist talking on a mobile phone.

They pedal, and do not seem to get tired. They often have their ears covered by headphones, a habit that in the urban traffic could cost them dear. They wear glasses, tight trousers, All Star trainers, and carry simple backpacks. Their hair blows in the wind. They can be seen at any time, even at night, in nearly all the bicycle lanes and streets of the city. They are studying, working, going to a yoga class, or on their way to meet someone. They ride because they like it; because the bus bores them, and they want to go by other routes. On arrival, they padlock their bikes, or leave them in the entrances of buildings. They have romantic faces; they are intellectuals, dreamers, or idealists. They know that things are not right, but they want to believe. This is where wisdom rubs against naivety. They glance stealthily at other cyclists, perhaps hoping to find someone like them. Generally, they ride austere bikes, without any accessory, other than a basket in the front to hold a bag. Not all of them are that beautiful, but the ride gives them a certain aesthetic flourish, which is becoming to them. They are in their twenties, and when they pass the scenery is no longer the same.

The Zen attitude helps us to shed all that is superfluous, all that we add to them in the name of... who knows what? Its tendency to simplify and not to impose anything is recognized by a minority of people. Despite the fact that Zen can bring another dimension to the life of anyone, in any circumstance and in any activity that they undertake, the majority see it from the other side of the glass. Zen also considers travel by bus or metro as possible ways to wake up.

No true master will do anything to attract or convince anyone. An aphorism, in tune with the paradoxical style of Zen, says, "When the student is ready, the master appears." The first part of the formula is the student: his desire to take the step, his predisposition. The second part (the master appears) is the result of the first: it is implicit, and lives from then on in the student.

I have to repeat as many times as necessary: riding a bicycle is not an isolated phenomenon, nor does it concern only those streets and avenues that have reached a point of saturation. It forms part of a series of transformations as a result of realizations. The authorities are aware that the incidence of motor vehicle ownership increases in proportion to the manufacture of more units, with the benefits and unwanted side effects that this entails. Theirs is a reaction more than a creation. The users think, *This is a freedom that is still possible, that does not happen because of some law but because people take the initiative.*

I tell a friend who is a hyper-cyclist what happened to me a while before with my client and what inevitably happens every time I go up the stairs with the bike over my shoulder. Does he fear that his employees will be infected? Or is it by the image of the not very serious editor that is advising him? Or is he worried for my life? No. It affects him, I think, to see me claim the freedom that I authorize for myself. To see that one of his peers gets pleasure from going back to cycling in the city, integrating it with his work, and above all, having fun. This touches a nerve.

Yes, it bothers him that I allow myself to do it. That I am not afraid to be different; different even among people who, like him, feel different. He feels confronted, through his body, by the fact that I use my body and not only theorize about the possibilities of it. I expose myself not only to taking a tumble but also to ridicule. Perhaps he feels the awakening of a certain wild nature that arises when the legs are moved and generate power from the low centre. Something very primal.

"When you release the animal," says my hyper-cyclist friend, "everything can start to fall away."

"What at one time was considered a rarity,
or disorientation, suddenly, without anyone
being able to explain how it happened,
becomes the most sensible alternative."
—Greil Marcus

In electronic music, they talk of a "boofer" effect that, for better or worse, creates a third source of sound between two speakers. In systems analysis, it is held that the whole is greater than the sum of the parts and something emerges from the interaction of these parts.

"More cyclists in the street means that there are more cyclists in the street," adds the boy who liberated the cars. That boy was on a closed stretch of road.

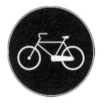

The City as Location

"This point of view [from a bicycle] —
faster than a walk, slower than a train, often slightly
higher than a person—became my panoramic window
on much of the world over the last thirty years."
—David Byrne

Those who have emigrated and return also see the city with other eyes. For those of us who live here, the façades are everyday backdrops, frames, and backgrounds, not protagonists. We get used to the idea that frontages become uniform, along with new buildings, shop windows, and advertising hoardings. We stop seeing the character of each place, house, street, corner, square... and what we see is flatness, the landscape made drab by our routine journeys hidden in buses and cars. We see with old eyes that do not want to discover.

For some years, I was forced to use the car a lot, and one or two times per week I had to cross the city in various directions. I said we are going to such and such a place, and the car went there alone, always by the same routes. My internal map was reduced to a series of rat runs, main avenues, signs, traffic jams, and queues. I barely knew what was there.

"Cities," points out musician David Byrne in the introduction to *The Bicycle Diaries*, "are physical manifestations of our deepest beliefs and our often unconscious thoughts not so much as individuals, but as the social animals we are. [...] Riding a bike through all this is like navigating the collective neural pathways of some vast global mind."

Seen from closer, not as an indefinite block of more or less uniform frontages, but as a diversity of neighbourhoods, the city becomes less anonymous, more friendly.

A house with a garden in front, a pergola, and a lady wielding a long-handled duster. I cannot avoid comparing this scene with all the anonymous and impersonal façades of the other buildings. The contrast is enormous. It makes me wonder about the choice—or non-choice—of life that each of us makes. It makes us pass through the city like people who are going blind and find themselves in a maze whose walls are so well known that they lose all shape.

It is not alienation, otherness, nonconformity, strangeness, insulation, or absurdity. None of the words that we used in the years before postmodernity sum up this impression.

In Zen, when meditating or when trying to meditate, thoughts and recurrent concerns tend to lead us by those circuits marked out by habit. The practice of meditation aims to drain the mind of content, to open us to other routes not frequented, to let the cursor roam free. Now and then, there are real surprises, and new ideas flash into consciousness that make you wonder, "Why didn't I realize that before if it was so obvious?" They were there all the time, but the mind's eye passed them by as it travelled the ruts it was used to. Crossing the city by bike and the surrounding neighbourhoods produces a different effect to doing the journey by car or bus. You are not travelling in a shoebox, looking through tiny holes; you are inside what happens.

You see the same thing from another perspective. If you go out cycling without a fixed route, and let yourself be guided by what you see, you discover that in certain neighbourhoods that you think you already know there are other neighbourhoods. Remnants of the old, new configurations, habits.

To ride slowly on a bike, with a vision less fixed on the place where you are going, or stopping before what amazes you, allows you to perceive details that enable you to grow. Great, small discoveries in themselves.

Open your attention to everything that happens, look without being attached, expand your vision, and see more: this, in Zen, is known as " full mental presence" (*sati*). The Vietnamese teacher Thich Nhat Hanh says that any act undertaken with full mental presence can be transformed into a rite as part of a ceremony. Clean the bedroom, hold a cup of tea, look out of the window... everything can be a rite, depending on the attitude you adopt when you do it.

The word rite has, perhaps, a too solemn connotation. Zen uses it so that the practitioner immediately understands that realization, or the expansion of awareness in a conscious way, is not an option but a matter of life or death. An awakening from the darkness of illusion to reality as it is.

To develop full mental presence may at first seem to be the same as to focus the attention, which means open yourself to experience, enlarge the lenses through which you see the world. Presence of mind is to be in experience and to see directly. Frederick Frank, in *The Zen of Seeing*, compares this with an eye that does not judge, moralize, or criticize; it only accepts. To accept is to see what is. When you do, this discernment emerges and awakens the third eye, and this sees that everything is connected.

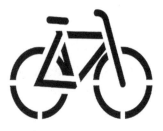

The Invisible Community

"To be one and to be part of a greater whole
is the same thing."
—Fred Donaldson

We were intruders in the traffic system yesterday; today we are flocks; and soon we will be a plague. Without talking and without touching each other, we multiply naturally. Associations are formed. Municipal authorities organize "bike rallies". They plot networks of bicycle lanes to cross the city from north to south and east to west, provide marked bicycle parking places, increase the number of public bicycles available, and create more pick-up/drop-off points. Security issues and road safety awareness are discussed, and some local authorities even finance bicycle purchase. Some small towns inland promote cycle touring days to draw attention to classic locations. The traditional bike shop returns to take its place among the shops in the neighbourhood. Film festivals are organized, in which the bike has some kind of role. The word "cycling" is no longer associated exclusively with racing and, with increasing frequency, the media uses the expressions "cyclist" and "cycling culture" to sum up the phenomenon.

In the etcetera of movements and activities that are emerging around the bike and urban cycling, some manufacturers now run simple mechanical workshops for children and adults to kick-start training. It is estimated that the growth will require 200 new professional bike mechanics each year.

"I never thought that this would be part of a revolution," a lady who pedals gracefully along on a small-wheeled bicycle confides in me discreetly. "What do I call my bike?" she says. "My Chiquita." "Come on, my Chiquita," she tells it often.

When two cyclists cross, they greet each other with their eyes, without diverting their gaze from looking forwards. A second. Sometimes a fleeting blink. They do not need to know each other. This minimum gesture is sufficient to confirm that they have something in common, then they continue, each on his own way.

Once, drivers of the same make of car who passed each other on the road, whether at day or night, signalled to each other with their headlights. Between cyclists—even if one has a very well-equipped bike and the other's could not be more simple and basic—there is a tacit recognition that articulates the feeling of belonging to the same movement. They do not need to put into words what they feel. At least in this one aspect, you know that other is someone like yourself. They have something in common. You know the other person has had the same inner experience, and he knows that it is possible to cycle in the city.

They may belong to different urban tribes, be of different sexes or ages, have contrasting idiosyncrasies and pastimes. They may be using bikes for different reasons. There is still a silent attitude, firm but intimate: *I'm keen on this. It is convenient. It resonates with a part of me.*

Beyond the fact that a bike is for a single passenger (traffic laws forbid you to carry passengers), using one has to do with a choice made by you and for yourself. Often in spite of the judgement, based on fear, of those around us.

Even if you ride with others, or amongst them, you will always be alone, and you will almost always ride without speaking. You think, and you let yourself think. Thoughts come and go and are interspersed with what you are seeing. There comes a point in time when you forget that you are thinking. When you stop talking even to yourself. Wherever his mind is, the cyclist makes the journey alone. He is a loner.

To be alone is not to be lonely, but to be with yourself. Without needing an answer or the presence of anyone else to feel you are in company. You do not fear that you will be considered unusual. You are able to stay peacefully in that space. More than that, you need times like this in your life.

Buddhists have a word that is used with increasing frequency in other contexts: *sangha*. This can be translated literally as "a community of practitioners". By extension: a group with a goal, vision, or shared belief. The members do not need to know each other, to meditate in the same *dojo*, follow the same teacher or line of instruction, or have the same level of realization. It is enough to know that the other person is on the same path in order to consider him a companion.

The value of this sense of community is that by feeling included, and allowing others to be included simply because of choosing the same path, the searcher or practitioner feels the solitude with which he begins each day to be part of a shared experience, and this enables him to transcend it.

To know that there is a sangha tells you that you are not alone, nor adrift in a society that tends to standardize and to divide rather than unite. An invisible group protects you and gives you the feeling of refuge.

The sangha of the urban cyclist reminds you that each one is part of that silent, self-selected network that today weaves through almost all the towns and cities on the planet.

To recognize the nature of whom you have in front of you is also to recognize yourself.

Buddhists press their hands together across their chests and incline the torso and the head slightly. This is how they salute the nature of the Buddha that is in the other person (*gassho*). The cyclist performs this gesture through the fleeting glance of interaction that he shares with another person that comes pedalling along. This outline of smile is your sign of Zen.

"Who are you saying hello to?"
"That cyclist."
"Do you know them?"
"No."

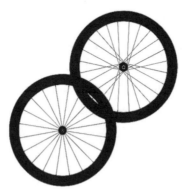

Blowing in the Wind

While the vast majority of cyclists probably do not know what dharma means (and often confuse it with karma), there is much of its meaning in their actions, no matter how insignificant they might seem in relation to everything that needs to be done in the world. It means: do the appropriate thing.

"Why?" and "what for?" are irrelevant compared with "how?" in whatever we do. Even more important is "from where inside us?"

Like every follower of Buddhism, initially they find it difficult to accept that many actions, in particular those of a social nature, do not arise from mere civic activism but are guided by a *force majeure* (dharma). Actions that are taken because it feels necessary, regardless of the results, the rewards, or who will benefit from them. Actions that may appear to be driven by our ego, but really respond to signals from a universal natural order.

Dharma also means "that which holds or keeps things together". By extension: sustain, sustainable, sustainability—concepts inherent to an ecological worldview.

Part II

I Celebrate Your Inner Bike

Doing It, Enjoying It

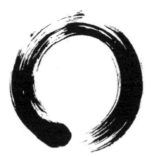

2

Riding

All the teachings of Zen are represented by the simple act of getting on a bicycle and starting to pedal. Keeping your balance and getting into a rhythm of firm smooth movements activates your brain waves. Einstein had the idea for the theory of relativity while he was riding a bike. Believe it or not, cycling is a route to the same kind of freedom that you get when you meditate.

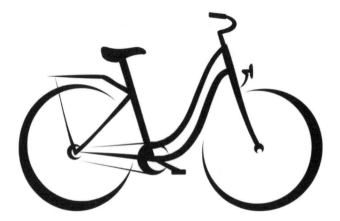

Pedal and Look

*"Give way. Or do not give way. Instead launch yourself
with sufficient decisiveness that whoever comes at you —
whether on bicycle or on foot, from the right or the left,
sometimes going the wrong way — gives way to you in a
negotiation that lasts only seconds, or even fractions of a
second, and during which only the beginner applies a
burst of acceleration or stops altogether. Almost everyone
acts with an equal amount of dexterity, either speeding up
or slowing down in such a way that the flow is always
changing its pace and never comes to a halt. A series of
hesitations, slight detours, and accelerations and
decelerations ensures that each time two trajectories cross
a collision is averted by a fraction of a second, or a few
centimetres (inches). To the uninitiated coward who
pinches his nose, closes his eyes, and jumps into the water
any which way, it looks like a great mixture of daring and
deference. Part of the skill of the native or the regular consists in circumventing the clumsy stranger; in anticipat-
ing their mistakes and abrupt stops."*
— Antonio Muñoz Molina,
"For a Basic Dictionary" *(El País, 15/9/12)*

Saturday morning. Between the shelves of a Chinese
supermarket, I believe I see a character out of a comic
strip in a Sunday supplement. He is short, with crew-
cut hair, and he has an expression of surprise on his
face. He is putting natural products into his trolley, and
in between them is his cycle helmet. He remarks,

"Using a bicycle has got something to do with all this, don't you think?"

Like cycling, Zen is not a method or dogma or religion. It is a way of confronting life, a non-verbal experience that allows us to establish a better contact with ourselves. It doesn't eliminate fear, anxiety, reactions, or force of habit, but it does show how these things cover up our essence.

When you ride a bike, you learn something about yourself. It is like the space in which you practise any martial art or artistic activity. The opponent is the activity itself, the street, our way of riding, and the discoveries that we make. To see the obstacles (concepts, words, false beliefs) that make us repeat old habits...

In Japan, the concept of art transcends aesthetics and the way to achieve a literary, pictorial, or musical creation... Art is the "attitude" with which the person performs an activity, whether artistic or otherwise. Art is what is done when you give yourself to the experience, beyond technical knowledge; when you let yourself go wherever the activity takes you. Art is an initial predisposition to a process that defines its own rules as it progresses.

In most Japanese martial arts, this attitude, encrypted in the suffix *do* (judo, taekwondo, aikido, kyudo), adds a sense of "way" or "path" to the activity—that is, a road to be travelled. It is not by phonetic chance that the art of arranging flowers (*kado*), and many other activities, ends with the same syllable.

The practical part of riding a bike is the method: how we do it. The idea of a path does not imply going towards a destination but what is discovered in the doing; by making contact with the way in which we conduct the activity. It is in the mental states that we reach through the practice. In the calm and precise manner that we make all movements, however insignificant they may seem to us. In the gaze that, at the same time, looks outward and inward.

If we consider urban cycling as a method, in the sense that Zen gives to any non-competitive sport or to art, it allows us to approach the experience from another dimension. To ride a bike without expecting anything, except the mere fact of doing it, is like putting yourself in motion in order to counteract a sedentary trend, or go to a particular place cheaply: to convert it into a form of introspective practice. It is pure Zen.

In the Japanese and Chinese traditions, the main objective of any sport or martial arts is not to compete and win; it is not taken as a chance to be better than the rest. Sticks and swords are not brandished to defeat an opponent: the certainty of defeating an opponent removes the necessity to have to compete with him.

These arts are not "danced" in order to create rhythmic movements or provide aesthetic enjoyment for others; the dances are practices that seek to harmonize the conscious, the unconscious, and the different energetic states of which we are composed.

Far away, in the cradle of Zen, the physical activities that Westerners call sports are considered rituals. They are respected—and honoured—as arts. The physical arts do not imply sporting ability, or mastery of the body, but rather have their own physical nature. The meaning is not looked for in the acquisition of skills but in inner exercises, whose purpose is to access the transparency, the alignment, and the surrender to the force that arises inside oneself when the will is unified with the movements.

In archery, a traditional sport in Japan, you are not trained to improve your accuracy but to achieve the natural release of the arrow. The arrow is fired and hits the target, not because the archer has his eye aligned with the arrow, the pull of it, gravity, and the target but because the archer is centred and in balance.

A Zen master of cycling would say: ride, ride. He would make his disciple ride a long way before saying another word. Perhaps he would be on a bike himself, behind, observing his pupil without influencing him, waiting for some signal that the huge flow of ideas through the disciple has begun to be diluted by its own inconsistency. When we begin to understand that it is something else that is required, the master may once again open his mouth: "Continue in that way, without looking at what I do."

In Japanese, practice (*shugyo*) is gaining capability, honing skills, training. Sanskrit combines two words that mean walking (*patti*) and front (*para* or *prati*). The Chinese, when they say *Xiu xing*, refer to the master, as master of himself, someone who completes, cultivates, studies, acts and, ultimately, goes. The Greeks' *practike techne* goes back to the idea of acquisition by the means of action. In English, depending on the context, to practise can mean to exercise, to learn skills through repetition and experience, to routinely perform some action or simply to do.

Riding a bike is so simple that the first or the second time you get on one, you ride it and forget that you are also doing an inner training.

In any activity framed as a means to explore and express the purest part of yourself, the concept of practice adds another meaning: the chance to make mistakes and to recognize signs in these mistakes. Why? To transform them.

If you do not see what you are doing wrong, if you do not accept your mistake, if you reject it, or if you try to combat the error as if it were an enemy, it will be difficult for you to transform it.

This attitude of accepting "what is happening as it is happening" is recognized, in the study of human behaviour, as part of a humanistic vision that is both ancient and, at the same time, forward-looking. It identifies a radical difference between change and transformation. A part breaks so it has to be changed before you move on to something else. That's fine for a machine, but how do you do the same with a personal characteristic? It is impossible to remove it and replace it mechanically with a new one. You can try to isolate it, keep it under observation under controlled conditions, or you can smother it as best you can and suppress it when it tries to reassert itself. However, in some moment when you are not watching, it can rebel and manifest itself in another form.

When we are in the right energy of acceptance, this leads us towards a more consistent and harmonious place, where we can admit that we all have certain personal features that we dislike (or which do not make us look good). We can then reach out to them with love.

Like true mystical practices, the theories of psychiatry and psychology also begin with listening to the inner voice, whose purpose is to teach us to discover that, beneath our self-destructive behaviour patterns or mechanisms to repress our essence, there lives a wise entity to which we should listen. What in the terrain of psychology is called the "unconscious", or the "inner child", does not differ too much from the Buddhist idea of "spirit" or "light".

Practice means to be completely yourself, here and now.

- Be fully yourself in this moment.
- Be completely one with what you do.
- Be completely one with all aspects of daily life.

In meditation, the fundamental operation to perform is described in several ways: do not initiate; do not start; let go; give rise to a thought, but don't hold it. If there is an objective, it is only to create a structure, a framework of discipline, to discover what is in the nucleus. Of each one.

The practice has no beginning and no end. The typical meditator, the black belt in any martial art, and the veteran artist know this. The cyclist who never ceases to practise knows it, too. That is why he does not complain and repeats the same routines as a beginner to integrate the internalization.

For those who grew up listening to the formula, "If you do what we recommend, you will achieve what you are looking for", the notion that training can take a whole lifetime may be hard to accept. Your head wants to make sure beforehand that some day you will be able to say, "I have got there". It takes a long time to admit that the prize was always there in front of you and is intrinsic to the practice.

A neighbour recommends his hairdresser to me. I go there one day, first thing in the morning. The shop is closed. I wait, leaning on a parked car. Two minutes later, a man arrives on a bike specially designed for mountain races. Shorts and lycra T-shirt, helmet, backpack, goggles, gloves, cycle shoes... He takes out his keys, raises the metallic shutter, and goes in without saying anything to me. I watch him go up to the mezzanine floor.

Shortly after, he reappears dressed in an informal way and says, "Please come in." In a mirror, I see the rear wheel of his bike, half-hidden by the stairs.

"Do you train?" I ask.

"Yes. I live 20 kilometres (12 miles) away. Every day I cycle in and cycle back. The car you were leaning on is mine; it stays here."

A month later, when I go back, he tells me that he may go and take part in a race in the mountains on the next holiday weekend. He gets out a map blown up from Google and studies the curves, ascents, and descents. He is still not sure if he can go. I ask him if he ever rides for the sake of riding. Those who train sometimes forget to go out for enjoyment.

He reads something out to me: "While I run, I simply run. As a rule, I run in the middle of the void." He looks up at me and shows me the cover: Haruki Murakami: *What I Talk About When I Talk About Running*.

"How did it go?" I ask him the following month.

"I didn't take part; it was too risky." Awareness of limit.

The Eternal Present

"When riding, the bicycle is where the bicycle is not."
—Transliteration of an ancient Chinese paradox

"How did it go?", I ask him the following month. "I didn't take part, it was too..." Images, abstractions, no words, the road to take, the time that the trip is going to take, what am I going to do there, remnants of what I was doing a few minutes before, a conversation or mental images, incipient ideas that ceaselessly get associated with others, emptiness...

If you could film what your mind gets up to when you go out on a bike, however attentive and careful you are, you would get a sequence like this.

Mental activity does not cease but, little by little, the movements of the legs, the energies that this involves, the vibrations that are transmitted through the handlebars and the seat, the wind on the face and arms, cause it to diminish or force it to coexist with other mental states, in particular with that rare state of attention to what happens "here", in the immediate now, moment after moment. Other thoughts—to "ride with your head elsewhere"—lead to a sense of egocentricism that makes some cyclists believe themselves to be alone in the street. The unexpected happens; the cyclist makes a sudden manoeuvre and falls. Greater presence: let yourself flow through the succession of present moments and this induces a floating sense of attention.

Be in the here and now, recommend sports instructors and spiritual teachers. This seems as if it should be as simple as walking, but it is not something that can be controlled. Willingness alone cannot accomplish it. It is not sufficient to resolve to put the mind "here" and believe that it cannot be moved. The chatter, the film, the trips to other places: they all come when you drop your guard and invade the conscience of the now. The mind is so used to this that it doesn't even perceive when it happens.

Although we want to remain in the present, it is our nature to always be wandering here and there, without consulting us. In addition, this precise moment is a permanent fugitive and, before we can tie it down, it is always another moment, and another and another. The problem is how to stay put in this continuity of "nows"?

A monk arrives in a village and enters a draper's shop to ask the location of the monastery. He hears the following dialogue between the owner and a customer:

"Show me the best fabrics you have."

"Everything here is the best. You will not find any fabric that is not the best."

While the customer steps aside to look at the material, the merchant asks the monk: "What can I do for you?"

The monk puts his hands together and says: "I want to stay and meditate in your shop."

Becoming aware of what we observe day by day while we are on automatic is the way into Zen.

When you pedal, the first thing that you perceive inside is that flat sound that the air makes as it enters and exits through the holes of the nose and mouth. If you are relaxed and follow it, you will find that it creates a rhythm. It doesn't matter if the breath is long or short, if there is room for more air, or if you exhale all that enters, when you begin to see with the mind's eye, it enables you to notice the areas of the body to which the air reaches.

Breathing is the best way to connect with the here and now. Yogis say that when we breathe in not only do we nourish ourselves with the energy of the universe (*prana*) but that energy is reunited with the universal energy that is in us. In fact, conscious breathing demonstrates how the mind/prana law of reciprocity works. Each emotional state regulates a particular type of breathing. Serene inspiration invariably accompanies similar mental activity. Short breathing cycle, agitated mind.

Even in the middle of traffic, you can carry out the

exercise of being aware of your breathing. It can be done for a certain number of breaths, say, 10 in and 10 out. Or you can concentrate on pedalling, or on complete cycles of rotation of each pedal. This trains the mind to stay calm in the middle of the crossfire between casual thoughts, wandering thoughts, thoughts of the past, and thoughts of the future.

It is best to fix your attention on how the flow of air enters the body, where it reaches, how it stretches the lungs, and then how it leaves and the places that it goes through. Before you get to the third or fourth cycle of breathing, you may notice that you are experiencing a passing thought, a small one, about what you are doing, the impossibility of keeping to the natural cadence, and what you have always been told about breathing. Or you may be presented with a mundane reminder of something you have to do: *Tomorrow the phone bill is due, and I must put money in my bank account.* Sometimes a sequence of wandering images appears, or a thought about some aspect of the route. You continue to breathe—counting six... seven...—and suddenly you realize that, despite concentrating on respiration, your mind is still paying attention to other things and taking its focus away from the air that enters and exits. No matter. That is what has to happen at that time. You have to realize that the mind is ungovernable, even for very short periods.

The first thing you discover when you begin to meditate is that the waterfall of divergent thoughts does not stop even for a second. This can be confusing and disappointing. It causes some people to doubt the effectiveness of meditation as a way to learn to concentrate.

It is not that thoughts disappear and reappear because of the work of meditation, or because the focus of consciousness is placed on breathing. It is your presence in the here and now that makes you aware. They were always there but before you didn't notice them. Therefore, this experience is in itself a sign of progress.

This realization is an approach to one of the most difficult moments of perceiving the trillions of seconds and thoughts that make up our life in this body. This is the paradoxical "now", about which so much has been thought, said, and written, and that can only be understood as flow.

To be in the here and now, in principle, is the ability to observe what we perceive, what we do, and what happens in the mind. Many spiritual practices stop at the stage of contemplation and use it as a first step in the training to learn how to observe without being disturbed, without judging, and without identifying yourself with what you see.

The difficult art of developing the awareness of witnessing does not tend towards indifference or passivity. It should be seen as a way of clearing forms of conditioning and prejudices that we incorporate subliminally and that distort our perceptions. What is there, in principle, *is*, and is neither good nor evil.

When you distance yourself from an observed object, it doesn't separate you from it; it integrates you into the experience.

Zen masters are more radical because they say that in reality "you" are that second. "What else can you be?" one of them pointed out. This second has no time or space. It cannot be the same second as five minutes ago. "How could it be?" continued the master, smiling. I am here. I am now. It cannot be the second that will arrive in 10 minutes' time.

The past only exists in our memory and depends on how we read the events in our lives. It has variations imprinted on it by emotional states that may differ from those that we remember. The past stays with us as experience, as karma (the totality of actions and their consequences).

The future never happens either, although we imagine it and locate it in projects and expectations. When it is on the point of becoming the present, the now consumes it and converts it immediately into the past. We can make forecasts but not live in the future. We are now. This foot that pushes the pedal. These hands on the handlebars. This crazy mind that refuses to be swept away by the Zen experience of being on two wheels.

We are this moment. This moment is all we have, although for us it seems elusive.

If neither the past nor the future nor the present exist as our senses conceive them (space and time would be an illusion: *maya*), there is never a now. And at the same time there is, because we live a succession of tiny moments. In the end, the ungraspable now is the only real time, and what you are aiming for in practice is to relocate yourself in the dimension of the permanent present.

It is always now.

"Here" can be anywhere; it is the precise place where you find yourself. The here travels with you wherever you go. Each one has his personal here in each present moment; the teacher smiles again and says, "Nobody ever can be in the here of another."

We leave work close to midnight. It rains, as it often does in London. Lola, a partner who rides a man's Hamilton bike with a double crossbar, approaches the railings where she has locked it and checks that the padlock is securely fixed to the chain. Without further ado, she goes into Leicester Square station. The next day, I wonder if it is not a risk to leave it all night in the street. "Yes," she says. "What if someone steals it?" "Then someone steals it," she answers. And she adds: "It's not the only bicycle."

When I return home after having done my errands, my mind is busy with all these questions. Another cyclist comes towards me from the opposite direction along the cycle lane. Even though I manage to avoid him and brake, we both end up on the ground. We apologize. We see that nothing serious has happened. Each continues on his way. I think, *Errors are part of the process. We can anticipate them; it is impossible to stay in the here and now all the time. That second of distraction could have cost me my life. The fall is an indispensable part of the journey.*

He reaches the traffic lights, standing on the pedals, with the idea of crossing if there is nobody coming from the side. As he can see that the cars are coming towards us at great speed, he stays there going around in circles in front of those of us who are also waiting. He is about 30 years old. Curly hair and Bermuda shorts with tassels. His bike is a disproportionate breed of free-style: it has large, wide wheels and vertical chopper handlebars. He does four or five decreasingly circles without losing his balance, and as soon as the light changes to amber, he sets off quickly, still standing on the pedals.

Make Contact

The part of us that gets on best with the here and now is the senses. While the mind sweeps towards the past and/or the future, sight, hearing, smell, touch and taste perceive the present as direct experience. When we appreciate subtleties in what we see, hear, inhale, and so on through these sensory channels, the internal dialogue (or chatter) stops, while attention is maintained on the contact.

One afternoon a few months ago, we were riding our bikes through a wood that surrounds the lake on a golf course. Chia suggests leaving the asphalt and going across the grass. We are going at the speed necessary to keep our balance when she says to me: "Allow everything you see to enter your eyes. Receive the colours, shapes, and movements of what is within sight." She is trying to tell me that what I see comes to me. My retinas receive without effort. I am not looking for these images; I simply allow everything that I perceive to enter through my eyes. I see the present.

Almost a minute passes between one thing and another. A strange harmony occurs: what I see seems to have stopped in time, and time seems to have stopped in what I see, my awareness included. A few minutes before, I saw only 40 percent of what I see now. I wasn't looking, and it passed me by. Rarely have I distinguished so many shades of green in the trees. Chia continues: "Now become aware of your ear canals." Each noise, each sound reaches me without me doing anything except bringing awareness to the receptivity of my hearing. I open myself to listen.

As I pay more attention, a variety of sounds and voices (from the closest to the farthest away) are evident, and I can even feel the vibration that they produce as they enter my ears. It is as if I have removed a filter that I had put between what I hear and what I want to hear. The "hearing threshold", it is called. This threshold is similar to other thresholds in other channels of perception. From this flow of background sounds, I switch to the foreground, and to Chia's voice, which adds another texture when she says, "While I see and hear, I also smell." I perceive the air and odours that enter my nose.

Breathing obscures the vision and what I hear. Just for a few seconds. Once the air has entered my body and the echo of its passage through my nose has subsided, I am able to appreciate more the details of what I see and hear. I am alert to irregularities in the ground, to other cyclists and walkers. A symphony of perceptual data connects me with the time and the place. She continues, "My available senses allow me to be this receptive." I can now feel my skin, the wind on my face, the cold in my hands, the heat in the clothes on my back, the sun, the shadows, my perspiration.

After a moment I become distracted, and I cannot help thinking that this exercise could be useful to many cyclists. Not as a meditation but, rather, as a training to calm the mind. Then she adds: "I see, I hear, I smell, I feel my skin, and I perceive my body, the movements that I make... Is there tension in my shoulders? Are my ankles doing anything? Am I tired? How is my breathing? Is there any taste in my mouth? Am I thirsty?"

These small personal "realizations" establish a more intense relationship between the outside and the inside. Another awareness. In my whole body, in all of my being, I feel that there has been a change of channel. Even my pedalling seems to be different. If all my senses are in this here and now, I am receptive. "I do not need to do more than to be in this present, and I am grateful," she says.

That high state of receptivity evolves for the rest of the ride. On other days, alone, I repeat the exercise.

Without Going Farther

*"The only Zen you find on tops of mountains
is the Zen you bring there."*
—*Robert Pirsig,*
Zen and the Art of Motorcycle Maintenance

Cycling is not an ancient art like archery, loaded with symbolism reflecting the depth of the Buddhist philosophy: the search for the inner centre through the finding of an external balance. However, each time you get on a bike, whether consciously or not, you open a door through which you can reach such an alignment. Riding a bike is like going through a swing door to get to that place.

Riding a bike is easy, but it is just as easy to get distracted and lose concentration. The first thing that archery teachers recommend is to bear in mind that it is not you who concentrates; it is your mental faculties.

The mind finds it easier to adopt rhythms that facilitate self-regulation and information processing in an automatic, unconscious way, allowing neural systems to take decisions on its behalf, rather than consciously contend with the ten million steps involved in performing even the smallest act. Speak, move the hands... If we were to perform all the operations involved in balance, pedalling, choosing the route, taking care with the traffic, and so on in a conscious way, we would surely fall over. It is like the story of the millipede that was asked how he was able to walk with all those legs: when he had to think about it, he couldn't do it.

If I pedal among the trees, I pedal with the serenity that is found among the trees. If I go between cars, I am going between cars, and a different attitude is needed; cars are part of our journey. I am not only someone who is isolated among the cars; I am in a relationship of man-bike-cars, and the mind perceives this. It is the mind that makes the connection.

Let what we see/perceive pass through the mind; let those images come in as they are, without any comment, or interpretation. As if you see them for the first time, and at the same time without being attached to their memory, that is, allowing the new to replace the old and for amazement to take their place instead. All this creates the kind of concentration needed to remain in a cautious here and now.

Despite all the risks, something works in the cyclist's favour: his eyes are usually above the level of the roofs of the cars. They can therefore see what is happening a little farther ahead, overtaking manoeuvres, and other stimuli around us. The downside of this field of vision is that it extends horizontally rather than vertically, and it does not take in the hands and elbows—the cyclist's lateral limits. The cyclist can forget that his width is dictated by the tips of the handlebars.

The majority of impacts and falls are not a consequence of something ahead. Blows to the cyclist tend to come from the sides. One of the most frequent hazards is easily overlooked when you want to advance down the space beside a row of parked cars or between two rows of cars waiting for the lights to change. Looking ahead can be a way of forgetting to watch out for the bumps sticking out of cars at handlebar height: side mirrors.

In general, cars leave you enough room to pass, but there is always one that narrows the space. To avoid breaking and losing momentum, we tend to pass between them, looking forward. A minor brush against a mirror makes the handlebar twist, thus redirecting the front wheel and throwing us onto the car. If the car is moving, it may knock you down.

To be part of traffic involves calculating the space required to pass such spaces, which must be at least 15–20 centimetres (6–8 inches) wider than the handlebars.

Archery teachers do not teach their students to look only at the target. No process is purely linear. The archer who masters his art opens a path within himself so that from the depths of his being an energy is directed towards the target. In its trajectory, the arrow reflects the simultaneity of processes or relationships of the archer. The method of letting yourself become a channel for this energy aims, first, at the centre itself:

to open a space within you so that this energy can flow. Without differentiating between what "shoots" inside you and the "shooting" of the arrow.

The cyclist who enters and exits this reality stays focused on what he is doing and on his environment. That is what happens. He travels without looking at any point in particular, but it is enough for anything to move in his surroundings for him to perceive it.

When we focus, our vision expands, which in turn extends our awareness. While it does not seem that we are concentrating on every detail, a pilot inside us is watchful. We activate a mental strength beyond logical thinking. Perception replaces reasoning. It is difficult to explain more, since this can only be experienced in the silence of the here and now. You realize what has happened when you get off your bike.

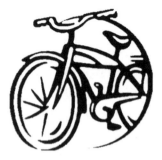

The Point of Balance

"Life is like riding a bicycle.
To keep your balance,
you must keep moving."
—Albert Einstein

By itself, without someone sitting on it, it falls over. You can lock the handlebars, give it a strong push, and let go. It will travel for a few metres in a straight line, like a coin rolled across a table, but when the force of the push peters out, the bike ceases to keep its balance and tilts to one side, the front wheel turns, and the bike falls over, with the wheels still spinning in the air. While you are waiting for the traffic lights to change, the same thing happens: the lack of movement obliges you to take one foot off a pedal and create a third support on the ground.

The balance does not come from the bike, or solely from being in movement; it comes from, and is maintained by, the rider: the person who propels it, balances on it, regulates its speed, and steers it where he wants to go.

Almost no cyclist thinks about balance, or has a concept of where that balance arises that he has managed to set in motion. Although it seems unbelievable, the balance, like the motion, comes from an imbalance.

When you take a step, you lean your body imperceptibly forward so that you leave behind that point of balance that enables you to stand on two legs and feet. This ability to fall slightly forward, using the highly controlled systems of regulation and balance in the brain, is one of the dynamics that enables us to progress. First one leg, then the other—your steps are made up of these small falls. Before you stabilize yourself, the other leg is already taking advantage of the forward displacement of your centre of gravity to take another step.

If you could locate a place in your body where you could tie a rope and suspend yourself in such a way that you could keep still in any position, you would have found your centre of gravity. If this interior point where all your mass is integrated is hoisted on a point of support, you are in balance.

When your centre of gravity is placed on a bicycle, in principle there are two centres of gravity: yours and the bike's. The line that connects the two points and meets the vertical of the two wheels creates the basic conditions for you to establish your balance when the bike is set in motion.

If, instead, you are running beside the bike, and you suddenly leap astride it and continue moving, thanks to the impulse you have given it, what sustains that balance is the imbalance that arises from putting your weight on the bike or pressing down first on one of the pedals and then on the other. This falling forwards onto the pedals, or the act of pedalling, not only makes you move but creates the right angular condition for the wheels to create a centripetal force (as with the rolled coin), giving the body the basic conditions for balance. The rest is the task of the hypothalamus.

To move to one side of any of the three centres of gravity—the cyclist's, the bike's, or both together—barely disrupts the balance. You do not fall off; the tilt is translated so that, without the need to move the handlebars, the bike turns. Every cyclist uses this effect without the need to understand the physical laws that determine it.

Children have stabilizers fitted to their rear wheels to help them find that master point without falling off. When they become familiar with it, they often move forward with the stabilizer wheels hanging in the air, without touching the ground. To describe the moment when fathers dare to take off the stabilizers, a biologist would say: he has found the system that causes the balance in his body. A Zen master would go farther: the balance had already entered his body.

The cyclist keeps his balance without thinking about it. Like walking, cycling becomes a reflex. When your centre is just right to keep you in balance, tubes in your ears tell you that you don't have to do anything; if it is more to one side than the other, this is automatically compensated for. When you lean over and stretch your head to one side to see if you can pass a car, your arms and legs make the bike tilt in the opposite direction and thus act as a counterbalance. The signal goes directly to the brain and returns as motor response to the muscles. The counterweight is not decided; it happens without our conscious intervention. Countless manoeuvres emanate from this double track of impulses.

In some streets, the bicycle lane is on the pavement. A local in the bar tells us that there are two schools near the end of the street, and every day he passes them on his bike. When the kids go in and when they come out, mums wait in groups on the pavement and almost all cyclists dismount or move into the street. A while ago, there was an incident that must have lasted two, three seconds...

"Suddenly, a little girl ran towards the car where her mother was waiting with the door open. Without thinking, I threw my body to the school side of the cycle track, but I could have run her over."

I ask him, "Haven't you ever seen the three signs that say: 'CYCLISTS, TAKE CARE'?"

"No," he answers.

Who performed this manoeuvre? It was an "I" that doesn't correspond to the concept of ego or to the role assigned to it by classical psychology. When Zen refers to the "I" it means the confluence between one's own personal consciousness and another expanded, universal consciousness, which it calls presence. An instance in which the mental processes leave the work to the frontal lobe, and we think without thinking in the non-thinking background or, as theories that do not separate mind and body have it, we think with the body, as a structure and as a process of energetic integration.

Consciousness is in the body. I am this body, which is my "I"; my being present passes through it. Immediate action is regulated by integrative mechanisms in the hypothalamus, not the frontal lobe. As we are not aware of these reactions, they seem to us to happen automatically.

Practice enables the cyclist to perform reflex actions—to receive sensory information and instantly produce motor responses, both when faced with familiar situations and new requirements. Practice trains us to react before we can think, *Now, what do I do?*

Why is it so easy to ride a bike? Because the mechanism for the necessary movements is based on laws similar to those that allow us to walk, and because stability is regulated by similar biological processes. Because the bike was conceived as an extension of the human body, it multiplies and maximizes the potential that we already have in ourselves.

Umberto Eco says that a mirror is really a prosthesis of the eye that allows us to see things that we could not otherwise see, especially ourselves. In the same vein, we could say that a bike is an ambulatory prosthesis that gives us new abilities, that allows us to extend what we are capable of, in terms of energy use, speed, and so forth. We can achieve feats with it that would be impossible with our own anatomy alone.

What makes us lose balance? None of the causes is a direct fault of the bike. All of them arise from some type of human failure. The reason may be not listening to the bicycle's maintenance needs; an unevenness of the surface over which the wheels pass; distraction (mental activity dominated by thoughts outside the here and now); flaws in the method of riding; or, most often, problems in behaviour encountered in urban settings, his own and others.

Whenever he was asked, "How are you?" the teacher would respond, "Very well."

One day a student wanted to know how he managed this. "Does nothing ever go wrong for you?" he asked him.

"Oh, yes!" replied the master, "but even so, I never cease to be well."

At first glance, it seems that the teacher had created a bubble, or a shell, around himself so that nothing could get through to destabilize him, so that he could always feel well. A state of denial and avoidance would be the diagnostic of any conventional psychologist. A smile painted on the face of a doll. Indifference... Another reading of the story is to understand that when the master says, "I am very well", he is speaking from the core of his harmonious self. If something is wrong outside that core, "there", he is still well. It is as if a gyroscope could maintain a state of awareness and remain in continuous balance: while the wheel spins, whatever position it is in, it is always supported on its axis.

Zen links balance with the concept of equanimity. Stay in the event, it says, without losing your centre or your calm. Eyes and ears unmovable before permanent changes. Without anything to hold on to.

The balance that the bike requires of us is dynamic: it changes continually and imperceptibly. The position that I am now in needs to be adjusted according to each situation. It would be impossible to keep my balance by clinging to it as if it were a railing. As in any activity, balance comes from an inner knowing "how", not from knowing "why", nor from any outside form to which I have to adapt myself.

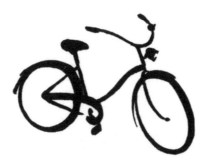

Let It Happen

"It is easy to feel calm when you are doing nothing,
The hard thing is to feel calm
when you are engaged in activity.
The calm in activity is the true calm."
—Shunyu

Eighty-five percent or more of your weight is supported by the saddle, and when you move forward, between 10 and 15 percent rests on the handlebars. When you get on a bike, you literally take the weight off your legs; you liberate yourself of your own weight and, as if that were not enough, you put yourself in a position to maximize the propulsion from your muscles (an imperceptible part also contributes to maintaining your balance). Something more: the circular movement that the pedals demand from you is a perfect fit for the articulation of the hip joints, knees, and ankles. The legs only need to overcome the resistance that your weight exerts on the points of friction in the axles. When pedalling you burn up 0.15 calories per gram per kilometre, at an average speed and without forcing ourselves. In contrast, when walking the figure is 0.77. In theory, cycling is a task five times easier than walking and requires five times less energy.

Cyclists and hikers get energy from what they eat and from the performance of their muscles. When you slowly exert a lot of force against strong resistance (for example, rowing against the current), or when you rapidly exert a small force without appreciable resistance (a punch in the air), you obtain a low rate of return. Between the two extremes, however, there is an optimal level of productivity that on a bike is achieved by constantly adjusting the gear ratios. That is to say, by adjusting the force and rhythm of pedalling according to the effort that is required, which depends on the wind, the slope, and the desired speed.

Pedalling makes you use the most powerful muscle mass in your body, your thighs, given that the legs work like cranks. At rest, you need some 150 watts to live. When a street slopes upwards, you have to overcome gravity and inject an amount of power proportional to your weight and that of the bike, along with the number of metres that you travel per second up the gradient. If the slope is 10 percent, and you weigh 65 kilos (143 pounds) on a bike that weighs 10 kilos (22 pounds), you need to expend 150 watts merely to overcome the extra gravity, if you want to go at 26 km/h (16mph). On flat ground, and at constant speed, the weight hardly counts.

A walker needs to raise and lower his body with each step he takes (practitioners of athletic walking try to limit this useless effort). In contrast, the cyclist is seated and always at the same height.

The cyclist gets an even greater benefit from the inertia of the bicycle. When you stop pedalling you continue to move forward as if the bike were in neutral. To begin with you travel almost at the same speed as previously, but then you slow down until you come to a halt. Once you get to cruising speed, you only need to pedal to maintain that inertia. At this point, 80 or more kilos (176 pounds) seem like three or four kilos (seven or eight pounds).

All cyclists take advantage of this aid to rest the muscles for a few seconds. If the road surface is not sloping, and you have to reduce speed for each corner, the simplest thing to do is to stop pedalling a few metres before so that you don't have to touch the brake. If the surface slopes, you can stop moving your legs and take advantage of the immobility to refine the ear and listen to the bearings. Awareness of inertia is rapidly integrated and automated, almost as soon you learn to ride a bike.

Zen redefines inertia as the river of life. A series of forces and currents of the universe that naturally flow inside and outside physical bodies, so that it is just a question of letting yourself be carried.

As the reeds lean where the wind blows them, life itself gives us a push, and our only task is not to resist. For the cyclist, this means not moving your legs more than necessary; not wasting your strength by pedalling more than you have to.

The German writer Herman Hesse was one of the first Westerners to understand this metaphor of the river of life. In *Siddhartha* (1922), Vasudeva, the ferryman, takes people backwards and forwards across the river and sums it up as, "just do what you need to do". If someone needs to cross the river of life, he sinks the oars into the water in the correct position for the boat to take advantage of the momentum of the current and sail to the other side. He doesn't give in to current or row against it; he rows with it. The correct effort eliminates what is unnecessary, the superfluous.

"I believe that you are the Buddha, because you have followed your own path," says Siddhartha, as he takes his leave of the Buddha.

"On a bike, everything seems closer," says Moisés, the husband of the neighbourhood chemist. For 30 years, they have arrived every day on their Japanese Mister bikes, imitations of old English bicycles. I meet him, too, in other neighbourhoods while he is running errands. Sometimes we chain up our bikes to the same lamppost in front of the bank. His has two square saddlebags that are very rare. According to him, they were his children's satchels.

That zero force that the pedals often asks of us, and the fact that the bike has a tendency to go straight, is associated with the Taoist principle of *wu wei*: "act only when you have to act." There is action in non-action. Creative calm. Play the game. To know that although we do nothing, we are always doing something or something is being done.

"Let it flow" is often confused with "complacency". Similarly, inertia with an "act by inertia", in the sense of going where the current takes you.

Wu wei alludes to doing without effort and maintaining harmony. This harmony is created by a sense of economy—doing only what is essential. Not to force yourself or resist natural forces; to act only when it is essential to do so. Make the correct effort in the right direction at the right time.

Wu wei does not imply not thinking; it means perceiving the order inside everything, the micro and the macro. To be prepared for what the path asks of us at each stage. Faced with conflict, triumph without a fight. In relationships with others, communicate without speaking. On the energetic level, attract without summoning. In everyday life, act without agitation.

Flow without influencing.
Live without interrupting other processes.
Facilitate without preventing.
Do not push the river.
Get rid of what is superfluous.

"Let everything be allowed to do what it naturally does, so that its nature is satisfied," writes Chuang Tzu.

On the bicycle, this does not mean stop pedalling but align your pedalling with other existing processes, to achieve and maintain a motion that is so serene that you almost do not notice it.

Without Intention

*"I ride a bike just for pleasure", many people say,
and they are being sincere.*

Take care, warns Alan Watts, with the word "pleasure", which branches off in two senses. The idea of
doing something just for pleasure, on the one hand, removes significance from it, making it seem trivial. In
that case, perhaps, instead of pleasure, it would be
more accurate to say: "I ride to live in the best way
possible." In another sense, says Watts, pleasure is far
from trivial: it means to do something in the best way
possible. This covers almost the entire range of human
activity. Whether you are playing a musical instrument, preparing a meal, playing tennis, carrying out
surgery, or fitting a dental implant, repairing an engine, weaving a tapestry, raising a child, laying bricks,
designing software—anything that you do in which
you deploy your technical knowledge and simultaneously commit yourself fully to the task in hand (to the
point that you stop thinking of everything else) engen-
ders a state of fulfilment. To believe that this pleasure
comes only from what you do or are able to do, is a
simple way to explain things, but it hides another,
much richer explanation: you enter a state in which
you allow yourself to be an instrument through which
energy can flow unhindered towards where it needs
to go. Afterwards, having allowed that energy to flow

through you, you are left with a sensation of pleasure.

The vital energy takes your body and performs the task without you realizing that you are doing it. A flow of energy runs through your neurons and cells without your intervention, and without you being able to interfere. At the end of it, recognizing the state in which it leaves you, you feel a mixture of satisfaction, relief, and emptiness. You are free for another thing; you are available.

The pleasure of having been the vehicle that provided such action leaves the body satisfied. You don't even need to be aware of this for it to occur.

Any ritual in which an activity is accomplished through involvement, commitment, and a striving for impeccability is recognized by the Japanese as an art: the art of calligraphy, the art of flower arrangement, the art of serving tea, the art of war, martial arts. Art does not imply, as it does in the West, the idea of a work of literary, musical, or pictorial art but the sense of mastery. Activity carried out with mastery.

A practice can be anything that is practised as an integral part of our lives, not in order to do it better, but to do it for its own sake. The artists of such an art do not do it to perfect their technique, but because they love what they do; and that is why they are the best.

From this perspective, the purpose of practising any art is not to find out who you are, as in psychotherapy, but to become your own truth; to be able to divest yourself of all self-delusion, pretence, and vanity, whether in relation to yourself or someone else. True art is not about satisfying the small ego; it is a manifestation of the "I" that transcends it and meets a "non-self".

Ignorance, or the error of perception, is manifested in the concept of "I" created by the human mind in the attempt to know itself and in the atavistic emotional attachment to that idea.

One of the first things that a new-born human being needs to learn by cultural imposition is the difference between "me" and "not me". He must learn to define his "I" as an immutable entity, always contrasted with the "not-I".

What the baby knows (but the adult has forgotten) is that no "I" can survive without what we call "not me". There is no separation between the "I" and the "not-I"; there is a continuity that blurs all limits. This is an error of perception; the other is the part of himself that remains hidden in the shadow of ignorance.

The Buddhist monk Walpola Rahula speaks of an "I" that emerges in periods in which perception is not dominated by any desire. It is experienced as an eternal and immutable realization. A centre that is witness to all events, exterior and interior. It is, explains, Rahula, the "I" of the "I" that "I am".

In deeply harmonizing with the experience of doing what they are doing (in a diverse range of activities), many people claim that they enter states similar to mystical ecstasy.

This notion of "not me", or of an impersonal "I" that can occupy our awareness, strikes a blow at the heart of Western beliefs and ideas about self.

This is possibly the most difficult concept to accept for anyone born and bred in a society in which doing is intrinsically linked to results, work or activity to effort, and enjoyment to what we receive.

In the specific case of cyclists, learning involves linking this experience to a sense of broader pleasure. It is to register with your senses and your awareness that "that" which is detached from the task is, at the same time, that which reunites you with it. To make way for energy is what gives us life.

Conscious Practice

> "This kind of freedom is precisely
> the opposite of 'just anything'."
> — Stephen Nachmanovitch

Sometimes I have no other alternative than to ride on the pavement. With the chain on the smallest rear sprocket and on the largest chain wheel, and pedalling as if in a race, I go almost at the pace of a pedestrian.

On one of these trips, a lady coming out of school with two girls walks in front of me. They do not see me, so from far away, I cry out, "Excuse me".

The lady pulls the girls close to her and says to me, "I'm sorry."

I answer, "Thanks", instead of saying, "It is I who should apologize."

The previous day, while waiting for the traffic lights to change so that I can cross a junction, I watch a girl on a bike pass over a new traffic island, go a few metres (yards) in the opposite direction, and take advantage of the still flashing red of the pedestrians' warning light to get in between them. There aren't any cars or buses coming the other way. She crosses and turns round. A car that comes out of the side street also turns with the amber light. The driver slams on the brakes and because of this, the bike scrapes past. The girl does not stop pedalling but continues on her way fast, as if nothing has happened, looking forward.

I do not blame her. I used to make similar manoeuvres, taking shortcuts where I could, going through red traffic lights when I could see that no one was coming from the other street—lots of seemingly small and unimportant breaches of the rules.

I justified myself by saying, "I am not putting anyone at risk." I did these things on impulse, as if the impulse was not answerable to any internal structure, but I still broke the law. I knew this, but I could not stop myself. I would just like to point out that the freedom that a bike provides also brings dangers, but there are ways to tackle them.

We urban cyclists apply the patterns of behaviour lurking in our minds to the way we use the roads. We see a gap between two stationary buses, and we go through it. We prefer to take one street in the wrong direction, with parked cars to both sides, leaving barely a gap in the middle for a car to get down, than to take two streets in the right direction. Sometimes, on corners, we do the same thing to pedestrians that motorists do to us: we do not give way to them. We take advantage of gaps in the regulations to break them. Flashing lights, red phosphorescent stripes, rear reflectors, a helmet just to go up one street... What are you talking about?

Even nowadays, it is difficult to tame myself: a part of me is triggered almost before I can take a decision. It tricks my sense of vulnerability.

Bike bad, good child.

It is not enough for me to know that I am doing something wrong to stop doing it. I'm riding along my lane but then, on impulse, if I can, I go wherever I want, as if I were a pedestrian.

Recently, I have been able to start modifying this behaviour by encouraging myself to accept that these are not only vices of the urban cyclist and that they correlate with other behaviours and reactions that occur automatically in my everyday life. These things, in fact, make up my personality.

Since realizing this—when I remember—when I ride my bike, I try to play the offender who offends against himself and perform the correct action to demonstrate its absurdity. There is a classical paradox: the liar who says "I am lying" contradicts the meaning of his words and doesn't allow his interlocutor to know the truth. In the same way, every time I put a foot down at a junction and wait for the green light before I proceed, or ride more streets than necessary so as not to take a one-way street in the wrong direction, or let a pedestrian cross in the middle of the street—I laugh inside and think of the double meaning of the verb "to perform" (carry out an action and represent a role). In truth, there is only one meaning: how we do something.

Once, I mentioned this private game to my close friend, who is almost a sister, Marcela Miguens, a psychotherapist who goes out on a bike with her clients. She sees what I do not so much as a performance as an apprenticeship. She says, "Imitation is a way to trigger the principle that you lie so much it becomes the truth."

When I was a teenager, I practised typing by copying extracts from the writings of Borges. One day, I began to change the words, another day the contents. You could say that I used his texts as if they were stabilizer wheels before I could bring myself to write by myself. After a while I stopped copying the words of the master and made up my own.

Riding as a "performer", doing what is right, gives me another relationship with cycling, and it never ceases to amaze me. Basically, I force myself to go slower, to relax more, and keep my mind more in the present that on thoughts of arrival.

When I am focused on doing the right thing, attentive to every circumstance, and at peace with everything that exists, riding a bike becomes something similar to what Zen calls the state of Equanimity. This is to be sitting in a quietness that does not depend on the body and the mind, but is instead a respect for the meeting between the I and the circumstances.

This attitude in itself keeps me awake. It disentangles old conditionings and allows me to own my reactions in any situation.

Wherever I go, nothing can stop me from using my freedom to exercise a sense of rectitude on the path. The freedom that a bike gives is like Zen—much greater than itself.

It is not the same kind of freedom that can install or maintain a certain political or social system, since a freedom granted can also be abolished. The cyclist breathes a freedom that cannot be revoked, or taken away. A freedom that flows in each one of us from deep inside.

Its objective is not moral (comply with the correct action), but to purify the mind until you can awaken to your own nature, which is simply to be. To what simply happens.

Whoever rides along the street (life) without breaking the laws, accesses that state of Equanimity, which flows from the condition of being aware. More than an ethic, it is an expression of love and compassion. These qualities have the ability to undo the conditioning that prevents us from showing a genuine consideration for others.

3

Wake Up, Energy!

*Each game or sport that we play is composed
of two parts: an inner and an outer.
Generally, we are taught to beat our opponent,
achieve the highest score, and be the best.
The inner game is about knowing our own nature.
We know this not through the eyes
but with the whole body and the mind.
It is not about thinking too much,
but about being surprised,
about allowing yourself to ride instead of pedalling,
and just seeing what happens. You find out by doing it.*

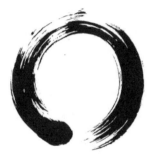

Aligning with the Bike

"The movement is done by itself."
—Zen proverb

Tuning, or "aligning" a bike, basically consists of calibrating the wheels; tensioning or replacing spokes; centring the wheels; making sure the brakes are parallel; adjusting the gears; lubricating the axle, bearings, cogs, and chain; maximizing the air pressure in the tyres; and adjusting any screw or nut that has come loose, whether or not it makes a noise.

Each time the bicycle man delivers my bike after maintenance, I feel it moves infinitely more smoothly and harmoniously and that makes it pleasant to ride. The inner tubes, inflated to their maximum pressure, jump at the slightest irregularity of the road surface but make for a firmer ride, without vibration. When the components of the bicycle are adjusted, they have less play; any space between them is occupied by the lubricant that allows them to rub against each other without roughness.

Everything is intended to reduce friction to a minimum; that is, to put the bike in a state of functional excellence (or of least resistance).

Alignment makes the bike more sensitive to contact and causes it to react to the least stimulus. I press a little on the pedals, and it picks up speed more quickly; any stone I run over has an impact on the handlebar.

A tuned bicycle implies less interference with the various actions and reactions implemented by the rider that naturally pass through its mechanical structure and through each of its elements. Good riding means not having to make any extra effort. I visualize several washers placed together. If the holes in the middle are lined up, so that there is no obstruction, a rod or cable that passes through the middle of them will not encounter resistance and will rotate or move with more ease.

Since I started to become aware of these issues, the image of the washers has been going around in my head, more as a hypothesis to test than as a metaphor. Does the same thing happen inside the cyclist? Does the energy flow in the same way as through the mechanisms of the bicycle? If I manage to align all the various parts of my body and the processes, will the forces involved—wherever they come from—meet less resistance as they pass through me, even though it is me who is producing them? If I manage to use only the necessary forces that each situation demands of me, avoiding any excess, am I attuning myself to the perfect alignment of the bike?

To achieve this, I need to learn to stay in my centre, through strategies adapted from other methods of self-knowledge. I am talking about achieving balance through calming the mind, loosening the tongue, relaxing the shoulders, paying attention to the breath, defusing the emotions, and letting go of expectations of a better performance. All this amounts to what Zen explains as removing the focus from the result to be obtained and concentrating on each tiny stage of the process.

Physical balance comes by itself, just like walking. Anyway, I begin to practise it through a basic relaxation technique that consists of doing a mental body scan of all of the muscles, one by one. I start with the feet and legs, listening to what they say; I try to move them in a graceful flexible way, as if a fluid is passing through them. The task is to do more than to loosen them; it is to become aware of the movements and let the energy pass.

In a broader sense, referring to the harmonization of our being with how we are and how we move in the world, humanistic psychology calls this "finding the centre in the alignment process". I don't mean to say that our life must rotate around an axis, nor that the axis should be the centre of everything, but we can go through any situation, however violent, without losing our internal balance. If our axis is not knocked off-centre, whatever position and situation it is in, it keeps all of our movements harmonious. Nothing takes you away from your centre.

The Japanese have an expression: "to have *zan-shin*"—constant concentration or continuous awareness. Whoever has *zanshin* is alert, aware, and focused, not only when playing but between games. There are people who are so connected with That, that they appear to be permanently uplifted.

These and other thoughts about how That occurs, both in the infinitesimally small and in the macro and in everyday life, came to me while I was looking at my bike or riding it. I felt I was "attuning" myself with it.

Beyond any theoretical elaboration, conscious practice expands my gaze and makes me see that the sense—if there is any—is not in the search for alignment, nor for my centre, but in the practice itself. The objective is not to ride better, with more fluidity, but to devote the time spent riding to the connection that is established through me, between riding and the That—sometimes called true, universal, or cosmic spirit, or Buddha nature, or the One...

Without intending it, That becomes a companion on my journey.

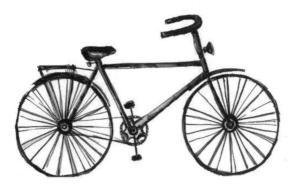

Learning from Learning

Every artist, whether Eastern or Western, knows that true art—which leaves the creator satisfied—does not consist in making movements "with art", but making them while being "invaded" by what he is doing, beyond what he knows and how to do it, so it seems to be this or that thing. Spontaneity, simplicity, impeccability, and what Zen calls "full presence of mind", and its own randomness is what makes art.

It is not a question of becoming a great artist on two wheels, but the nearest thing to this quest is the Chinese concept of *xiu xing*: to gain mastery in the sense of learning from learning.

It may sound presumptuous to talk about the art of riding a bike, when it is such a simple thing to do. The point is precisely this: to find the door to a cosmogony of correlations in something small and even routine and thus transcend the mere fact of riding. As in any process of energy, or in the transformation of energy into something else, there are aspects that go beyond rational understanding.

The majority of cyclists would throw their bikes at me, if I told them that when they get on and started pedalling they are setting off in search of their inner selves. Or that the force they exert on the pedals is not only their own. Or that an ethereal hand sustains us from a place that is not above, below, in front, behind, or in any direction, but is everywhere at the same time, including inside us. Or that in every moment the voice of the eternal is resonating within us. However, there is something of this when muscles, mind, and spirit unite to create graceful movements through space and time. Everything we do is synchronized with a whole greater than the sum of the parts involved, and goes beyond the mere fact of doing it.

It is an expression in harmony with a greater energy.

Sitting Within Your Core

We are used to thinking that strength arises from the muscles, that we regulate balance with the hands placed on the handlebars, that when we are tired our hearts pumps faster and that our minds decide what to do in any situation. On the every day level, these assertions can be taken as valid, since nobody needs to know much more than this in order to cycle. However, this concept ignores the element that connects the parts and their functions: the continuous flow of vital energy.

More than decipher the properties of this energy (known as *chi* in China, *ki* in Japan, *kundalini* and *prana* in India and *baraka* among Sufis), what we are trying to do is to facilitate its flow through the *hara*, the energetic core located in the abdomen, towards the rest of the body.

Tai chi chuan attempts to translate this ethereal rhythm into movements. By stimulating convergence points, acupuncture seeks to open the way for that energy to circulate better via the meridians that it considers as associated with each organ. Despite being considered a martial art, the goal of Aikido is to re-channel the subatomic particles of violence that arise inside each person in an assertive way and re-harmonize this energy.

Where is the enormous strength of sumo wrestlers situated, and distributed from, if not their large bellies? There is an area (a vortex, to be more graphic) in the middle of your body that feeds and links to the rest. It is located two or three centimetres (one inch) below the navel, where yoga sites the third *chakra*, the Chinese the *tan tien*, Sufis the *kath*, the Japanese the *hara*, and where any well-intentioned Westerner would place the body's centre of gravity. It is believed that the fuel needed by muscles to extend or contract (whether we are still or moving) flows from this point.

The Japanese also call the hara, *kikai tandem*: *kikai* being ocean and *tandem* energy field. As with the ocean and a field of energy, this processing centre is not a material palpable structure with a stable configuration. Modern physics uses the term "field" to cover the nature and role of phenomena, beyond their form and any type of anatomical description. Through this vision, we meet the Taoist concept of void (*ku*): the living vacuum where energies are undone and reconfigured in a permanent dance. Rather than talking about particles that pass through or compose it, the conscious mind can only get close to this centre by considering it metaphorically as a gas: a stream of "dematerialized matter" in its tiniest form that, for all its lightness, carries in it the *élan vital*. A nothing in which everything is contained; an elusive something that changes shape and rearranges itself in every moment. Any movement that we make reshapes the flow.

The *hara* does not operate as a gyroscope, and we cannot use the will to control the energy that arises or passes through it. Masters of martial arts only seek to learn to be aware of their potential as receivers, regulators, and distributors of these energies.

On a steep hill, you cannot generate power from your belly, but you can relax it and keep it relaxed, so that the energy that reaches your legs allows them to move with the least possible wear. In this situation, try to free the abdominal region and send air towards it: you will notice the lubricant effect on the joints and muscles of the lower limbs.

Those who work with the hara say that it doesn't allow itself to be known, only to be recognized. All the new information that enters (for example, a suggestion to straighten your spine) is based on the notion that what we do or believe (the mind focuses on the spine) does not come into a blank space.

In transcending the material dimension, the hara acts as an interface between the physical plane and the energy field, in which the life of the universe includes each of us. To act from the hara involves much more than an awareness of energy and its location; it points to a gradual process of recognition, openness, and re-union with the essential force.

The Japanese, who have incorporated the concept into everyday language, give the word a very broad meaning, that goes from "a state of being" to a stage of "maturation" on the journey towards awareness, that we are part of something bigger.

They were also the first to link this inner attitude with physical posture.

When they say that someone is "not in his hara", they do not just mean that his belly is compressed and his chest inflated; they "read" from his posture that he is disconnected from his axis, his centre of gravity. This, of course, creates physical tension but also energy loss and a sense of "not being centred". The emphasis on the individual self over the natural order is considered one of the origins of the physiological and psychological illnesses that afflict the modern world.

In the second half of the 20th century, the concept of the hara began to become familiar in the West. In part, this was because of the popularity of Japanese martial arts but, in a wider sense, it was because it speaks of the search for primordial unity, coupled with the emergence of a new paradigm in which body, mind, and spirit (awareness of universal life) are considered to be interdependent entities and expressions of the same energy that unites them with the order of nature.

In this regard, what Zen is trying to do is to reconnect the mind that tends to separate things (dualistic thinking) with the notion that opposites are complementary. There is not a world of acquired knowledge and another of intuitive knowledge. There is not a physical reality separate from a mental reality. There is not an exercise for improving technique and performing better (know how "to do") and an exercise that transforms you inwardly (know how "to be"). There is not a down and an up. There is not an "I" and that which is not me. There is not a relaxed immobile belly and another capable of acting quickly.

Learning is to move from a vision of antagonistic and contradictory opposites to a vision of primordial unity.

4

Man – Bike – Way

The ego is not left behind; it is nowhere and everywhere.
Your face, body, and the movements you make with your
legs pass through the air, ignoring the barrier between
yourself and the world. Cars and concrete,
the crazy urban beauty, your going forwards,
all dance together towards a single destination.
The poet and cyclist Gary Snyder wrote:
"The path is what happens—it is not an end in itself.
In order to walk the path, you have to become the path."

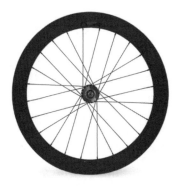

Awareness Beyond Words

> *"I went and came back. It was nothing special."*
> *—Su Dongpo*

I have never managed to recapture with the same intensity the sensation I experienced by the waterfront 30 years ago, as described in the first pages of this book—of nothingness, absence, forgetfulness, lack of thoughts, and of an emptiness that "wakes me up to the facts" (*wu* in Zen).

It has taken time for me to understand that it is the very desire to understand that prevents it from re-occurring. It only lets me evoke it after the event, never during.

At other times, many more than I remember, I may have had the same sensation in which I forgot everything I knew with regard to that wonderful feeling. Like millions of cyclists in any part of the planet, I lived the experience, or the experience lived me.

Almost every person who meditates at some point asks himself, *Who is inside me when I reach a point at which all thoughts cease? Where there seems to be nobody, not even the echo of the thoughts that have stopped? There is nobody to witness what has happened in that void.*

The Upanishads, the sacred books of Hinduism, leave no doubt. They state that if someone meditates, and he hears inside himself a "Yes, it has happened", or if someone listening to a teacher says, "Yes, I understand", you can be sure that in both cases "That" has dissolved.

The closest answer (neither the least illusory, nor the most real) would be to reach silence without wanting to understand. Just to know that the "That" may have visited you and nothing more, leaving behind its ethereal lightness.

Forget Your Identity

When you meditate, and you make the slightest effort to keep your mind blank (or black, or in a state of nothingness), you are introducing dualism and artificiality. Nothing is more counterproductive when trying to reach that state of absence than to be alert, watching for it to happen. When I cycle and suddenly arrive where I am going, almost without noticing the journey, I try not to look back in search of answers. I do not want that state to establish itself as a thought-form. I run a similar risk now in writing about That.

The sensation of absence has nothing to do with what our Western culture means by absence: lack or passive waiting. In the state of no-mind that occurs on countless occasions (not only when cycling), there is a strong sense of presence. The mind less dominated by thinking remains alert to everything that happens, whatever that may be, and to messages from the body.

Some people call this process "integration". By this, they mean setting aside the differences established by the mind, thought, and language and, instead, capturing the flow as a whole—a flow in which the harmony of the parts creates a single interrelationship.

Zen comes to the same thing, but by another route: it comes from understanding that the self, the little man through whose eyes I look at the world, makes me believe that I am separated from what we see and puts up barriers, both inside and outside. If I think that what I am witnessing is not me, or that it is alien to me, I establish a division between me and it, and it is this division that sets me apart. When the Zen speaks of separating yourself from your identity, it is pointing out that "I" insist on convincing myself that the only thing that counts is my perception.

When I stop thinking that the outside is something separate from myself, it does not disappear; rather, it expands—it transcends the borders established by the edges of things and fuses with them.

The mind's eye separates things, events, and facts and conditions us to see them as separate entities. In the natural order, all phenomena, both physical and abstract, are in relationship within the whole.

When Zen suggests that you observe your mind, it does not do so to disassociate you from the experience. On the contrary, it seeks to link it to you in a different way. It wants you to see where the lines are that separate one thing from another and separate you from them without the parameters of your "I". It is also trying to tell you that the self is another element of the assembly.

Consciousness frees itself from forms. It dis-identifies itself and becomes a presence.

Any cyclist who has ever experienced this absence in the flesh does not need any argument to explain the sense of awakening. When pedalling, it becomes evident that he plunges into the same substance that surrounds him and that his vision is taken over by a capacity to become one with everything he sees, beyond what he sees. He perceives himself joined to something infinitely greater than his body, his consciousness, or his language. It is not an immensity in front, behind, above, or below; he sees it everywhere he looks. Something is there, at that moment, and it appears in the same as eternity might manifest itself.

I do not know what is,
only that it is.
Whether I understand it or not.

Little by little, ideas and thoughts begin to fade, and consciousness is liberated from its normal neural pathways. Mental activity becomes a field through which waves without content flow, or waves with self-generated content originating on planes that ordinary consciousness does not control.

The mind does not stop its activity. Some thoughts come and go, but the mind adheres to none; it sees them pass. This random parade is enriched by images that come and by responses generated in the mind; it cleans the mind and leaves it in a state of "availability". Openness. Order. Positioning. It seems that we are not thinking of anything; as if the mind or the self are not there.

The idea of absence corresponds with the emptiness (*ku*, in Japanese; *sunyata*, in Sanskrit) so familiar to Zen.

The emptiness that is in form, and the form that is inside emptiness. When you understand this reciprocity, you acquire another perspective on interior space and everything it does. The cup is the cavity into which you pour hot tea. Action develops in inaction. The sensation of the absence gives rise to other states in which That is seen through This.

When the commanding ego gives way to the void, new powers have the opportunity to come into action. Even if you think you are making an effort, the actions seem to occur by themselves. When the old habits are suspended, new powers can go into action.

It was difficult—is still difficult—for my mind to accept the idea of emptiness as something substantial. I still refuse to accept that the self exists within something greater, without any centre, called "not me", and that the only way to possess something is to be able to release it.

On my journey, I have sometimes thought that the most appropriate word was "give", but in the verb "offer" there is also an underlying sense of intention. It is as if I was thinking, "Ah, what a good boy. He is making an offering for the sake of his karma!"

Buddhism uses the word *satori* (awakening) to refer to those moments in which we are led by the personal ego and act as interpreters and instruments of a fundamental cosmic power. In practice, *satori* does not exist; it is something and nothing at the same time. True awakening is unconscious. When we are aware, it ceases to be *satori*.

"If *satori* means waking and understanding, then I have had *satori* many times," wrote the master Taisen Deshimaru. "But this is not what *satori* means. The true *satori* is a return to the normal, original condition of the spirit."

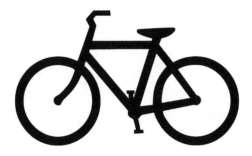

Everything Is as That as It Can Be

You pedal, and the minutes pass without you realizing, because you are in the present moment, which advances and moves as if following the front wheel. Time and space are the same.

The eyes look inward and outward at the same time. They may seem indifferent, but they are taking in information. The mind stores graphic memories. Its intention is not to discover anything in particular but simply to keep the attention afloat. This way of understanding reality takes the cyclist closer to the contemplation of the mystic than to the screen of a video game.

When it leaves you, the "I" does not disappear; it integrates into the process by a logic that it is difficult for Westerners to accept—by not being there, scanning everything, it is more integrated into the whole.

A harmonious simplicity governs the interrelationship of the parts and aligns us with a greater scheme. There is no difference between "I" and "myself" and going forwards on the bicycle.

On a bike, the body seems to lose its weight and the mind to expand its consciousness.

It comes; it goes. Something of That continues underneath.

When I perceive the bike between my legs as an extension of That it makes me forget my body. First I forget the processes of analysis, prognosis, and decision that are carried out each second. Then I forget that there are two separate entities, one alive and the other functional. I forget the five points of physical contact that join us. I forget that the wheels are supported by the road surface, and that there is an infinity of other beings around me. Body, bike, and road fuse, and my mind is out of time, out of the journey, and outside the body.

If there is an "I" present, it is that of experience.

There is a story circulating on the Internet that is probably apocryphal but is nonetheless eloquent. A Zen master sees five of his disciples return from market, riding their respective bikes. When they arrive at the monastery, he asks them why they went by bike.

The first responds, "I can carry this bag of potatoes on my bike. I am pleased that I didn't have to carry it on my shoulders."

The master comments, "You are a clever boy; when you are old you will not have to walk bent as I do."

The second responds, "Master, I can watch the trees and fields go past when travelling on a bike."

The teacher says, "Your eyes are open, and you see the world."

The third responds, "When pedalling, the universe penetrates my mind."

The teacher says, "Your mind will work as perfectly

as a wheel that has been newly balanced."

The fourth responds, "Pedalling, I feel in harmony with all beings."

The teacher nods, "You are on the golden path."

The fifth student answers, "I ride my bike, just to ride my bike."

The master sits at his feet and says, "I am now your disciple."

I ride my bike just to ride my bike. It is like letting the arrow itself decide when the finger must release the bowstring. The fundamental attitude to everything that can be understood as practice has to do with "letting it happen", "don't search", "not trying to reach the unknown through the known", "clean the mind of all illusions"... and just ride in order to ride.

"Practice is an endless process of disappointments," says Edgardo Werbin, a doctor who specializes in emergency medicine, a semiotician, and a Zen master. "Everything we achieve disappoints us in time, and that disappointment is the master for the first four disciples."

If you wake up at three in the morning asking what it is all for, what is the point of everything you have accomplished and all your thoughts, a Zen Master would tell you the same thing as Edgardo. It is in these moments that the wall of dualism dissolves, and we see that happiness and despair are not so different, and that emotions that seem to be opposites—enjoyment/depression, jubilation/misery, good mood/bad mood—have something in common: they are products of our way of seeing things. The illusion is that which makes us see in this way.

The mere fact of considering the possibility that this is true seems to make everything, including life, robotic, repetitive, neutral, and samey. This feeling of boredom is another teacher, say those who have been on the path for a long time.

Who is it who is bored, if I am not the one who is beyond these emotions? He who slowly learns that every moment is new, not the same as already lived in the past and is repeated. Each time I brush my teeth, it seems the same as yesterday, but it is a new session of teeth-brushing; each time I go out on my bike, it is a new departure; each time I concentrate on pedalling... Zen poets use the metaphor of drops of dew on the grass each morning. The same drop that falls from one leaf to another is no longer what it was.

The awareness of here and now that moves from moment to moment, without comparing, without judging, without condemning and, if possible, without conceptualizing is also a silent drop of dew.

Silence is not to ignore the experience of emptiness; it is not to name it.

Silence is to listen and to allow yourself to look with new eyes, if possible emptied of what you already know. With the awareness cleared of memories and without using words. To see what is ahead and to the sides. To see what is as it is.

This attitude, which is at once very difficult to adopt and at the same time very simple, allows you to ride a bike with presence. You are thus able to slip from moment to moment, and faced with each situation all you can say is, "How wonderful, how wonderful." Or you say nothing at all and continue to perceive it as a subject and as a witness. "A second self who is able to watch with dispassionate curiosity," as William Styron puts it.

The state of enjoyment and happiness that cycling produces makes your cells smile. I cannot find a better verb to describe this feeling, and I imagine them bowing their lips upwards.

The inner smile reflected in the faces of the majority of urban cyclists speaks of the feeling of freeing themselves of the self and of the past. Every moment that you live on a bike, however repetitive it may seem, brings to the awareness and the body the amazement that each present moment offers. Always.

That is the invisible experience; the direct experience.

The rest is pedalling, observing the breath and trusting, even if you do not understand in what, or why.

It would seem that there is no other secret.

Daily Life as a Journey

In his book *Be Here Now*, Ram Dass (Dr Richard Alpert) gives some guidelines for maintaining perspective on the spiritual path, and these can be adapted to the preparation of the mind of the cyclist. As there are no goals, says Ram Dass, neither are there any stages.

When you pass the initial euphoria of any practice (in this case, non-competitive cycling), and the novelty begins to wear off, the actual learning can begin. To progress further requires abandoning the idea of perfection. Then you start to see with clarity the endeavour in which you are engaged.

Sometimes, you may experience a total calm, as if the learning had been paused and you are floating flat on a plateau. It is impossible to go back; the journey is irreversible. To stay in this emptiness, without asking anything, makes it into a contentment.

Every cyclist knows that pedalling in reverse does not make the bike go backwards. Once begun, the process of riding a bike does not come to a halt by us getting off; it only appears to stop from the point of view from which we contemplate it. This thought is an obstacle.

It is more likely that you have periods in which you seek one thing and in others that you look for something else. Do not expect revelation, recommends Ram Dass, since the less noticeable it is, the more transparent it becomes.

Buddha also seems to address the cyclist when he refers to the way, or path. He says that for each person, the path is the path of least resistance. It leads towards an encounter with the truth, with inner knowledge and a union with the One. A state of equilibrium that a human being can attain when he understands the laws of right living. It is based on the equanimity reached by transcending the "I" and being able to discriminate between the attractions that the world of form exerts on us. For Buddha, these attractions (or distractions) imprison the awareness and separate us from the spark of That, which is in each one of us. Buddhism and Taoism offer instead an attitude that they call the "middle way".

No bike manufacture claims—at least, not yet—that their models will carry you along the path or help you access higher levels of consciousness. By not saying it, they seem to take for granted a set of universal premises valid for all types of riding: the way gives no promises; you have to set out on it without expectations; it amounts to a progressive forgetting of yourself; and the energy is revealed gradually. On some stretches of the way, energy surrounds you and makes you realize the value of impersonal, silent, and invisible action. On other stretches, it demands receptivity, patience, solidarity, persistence, and courage from you. It always reflects the rider: if the bike goes fast, I go fast.

"He was pedalling very slowly, because he was carrying a bag of freshly harvested oranges on each side of the rear wheel and another on the handlebars," Ryúnan Bustamante tells me about a member of his dojo, Ermita de Paja. "The road was opening in front of him and closing immediately behind him. Like an epiphany."

Nowhere

> *"As a boy, I once chased the end of a rainbow*
> *on my bicycle and was amazed to find*
> *that it always receded."*
> — *Allan Watts*

To ride a bike, just as with any search for a broader sense than the usual, does not seem to lead anywhere. It is the most Zen thing that can happen!

Practice is only the way that you go, and the best thing about the way of the bicycle is that it never ends. The "I" that I know is never the "I" that I need to know. If I am fortunate, the destination point will always be two kilometres farther away for each kilometre I travel.

The dominant trend for so many followers of rationality and Cartesian logic is to think that to get somewhere we must "go towards it", in the right direction. We travel so many kilometres in search of something that is so close that at times we lose perspective and think we have gone the wrong way. Why is it that we can't accept that detours are the way?

To go far means to return. My mind is passionate about this and other phrases written by Lao Tzu. I write them down. I interpret them. I associate them with innumerable situations. I repeat them aloud, but my subconscious resists processing them.

The awakening happens through shedding things. You cannot even look for it—when you find it, it ceases to be.

What can cycling give me? The possibility to shed this deeply rooted belief that I am separated from the whole.

What seems to be a separation is what connects. The mind draws the lines; it makes gaps between molecules. There is not a person in one direction, a bicycle in another, and a road in yet another, and traffic on all sides. There are molecules that make tai chi movements together with other molecules that are moved along with others, and so on beyond infinity.

"When you forget yourself, you are the universe," pronounced the master Hakuin. It was not another of his famous koans. He said this only to help his disciples understand that learning is not a question of incorporating something they lack but of recognizing what is superfluous and prevents us from getting to what he has (or is). An innate capacity lies dormant in each one of us, like a snake coiled upon itself, ready to unwind itself and show our nature to us.

To ride a bike in a natural way is to withdraw control from the "I". Then you can let yourself be propelled and guided by the flow of chi, hara, your breath, and that full mental presence that appears when you allow the energy of That to pass through your body, the components of the bicycle, and the journey you are on. That flow also transforms each moment into nothing special. It doesn't need understanding; it is simply riding a bike.

A man of about 60 years old, well preserved, is sitting on a bench in front of the lake. Arms stretched on the back of the seat. Legs raised and supported on the cross bar of a BMX, from which the paint is peeling away. He says, "Why talk of the losses that I have suffered over the last year? Here, as you see me, I feel very relieved. We remain together, facing the mirror of water. Melancholy is incompatible with cycling, my friend."

Part III

Rules of Experience

Care, Meaning

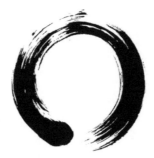

5

Right Riding

Function determines the practice.
Speed is associated with success,
and impeccability with wisdom.
What you do is how you do it.
The traffic regulations exist to protect the rider.
The freedom that a bike gives is part of a larger pattern
that connects you with those who go on foot
or in motorized vehicles. Whoever does not interact,
puts everyone at risk, particularly himself.

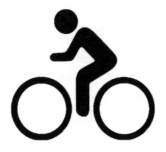

*"When we are fully on one path
we are indirectly preparing another."
—Ryúnan Bustamante*

Transformations only happen when we gradually free ourselves of deep muscle habits and replace them with others more suitable to the task. The body operates as an integrated whole during its operation and never as a series of disconnected parts.

Start by focusing on some aspect of the way you are riding your bicycle and this will have the effect of bringing other parts of the body into alignment. For example, if you pay attention to how you breathe, you will notice that your consciousness moves through your body with more ease, warns of any forced movement, and indicates some difficulty that you would otherwise ignore.

If you concentrate on the way in which you pedal and begin to recognize and eliminate inadequate muscular work, you will also become aware of efforts made by other muscle systems that are generated at the body's expense and contribute nothing to the forward movement of the bicycle.

There is no perfect way to ride but there is a way in which your individual behaviour and the actions you make resulting from it are better integrated and interfere less with your natural manner of riding.

From the moment you press down on the pedal and begin to ride, you enter a state in which you are fully aware, and at the same time you feel or are being carried by the action itself. Body and mind cease to be two entities that travel on different paths. If they are two, it could be said that each is aware of the other. In truth, they are a whole infinitely more interconnected than the mind can conceive or the body perceive. There is no word to describe this connection.

Riding a bike the Zen way, you do not think about what you will do when you get to your destination. Nor about how happy you are that you are not squeezed like a sardine into a bus. Now that you are pedalling, to think or worry about other things—about things you should do, or that could have been done, or could do—is to escape from the moment. It is a waste of energy.

Soon after you start to ride, with the mind occupied by the dialogue between legs and pedals, thoughts tend to disappear, the mind relaxes, and cycling becomes greater than the sum of its parts involved.

Pedalling

At first sight, it may look as if all urban cyclists ride in the same way. If you look more closely, however, without dwelling on the model of bike or the posture adopted by the rider, you will see that there are significant differences in the ways in which cyclists move their legs and feet. Some seem to carry the action of pedalling to the whole body: the torso moves up to the shoulders and the head rocks, as if in time to a piece of music. They ride with unnecessary tension and exaggerate their movements, as though they were working their leg muscles as if their lives depended on it. Others ride leaning back, as if driving a racing car.

In contrast, some cyclists move so smoothly that they don't seem to be making any effort to power the bike with their legs—they look as if they are riding without riding. Their movements come from the waist and have a natural sense of harmony; the leg muscles deliver the force necessary just to maintain the speed. A cyclist who rides in this way has a loose belly and, despite carrying his trunk in a relaxed way and his shoulders loose, he sits firmly on the saddle. He sits. He is not bent, and he does not push his chest out; instead, he is erect, which is not to say stretching upwards but centred on an axis.

He displays a centredness that arises from truly balancing his weight. He travels without haste, as if he has infinite time to cover his trajectory and does not doubt that he will arrive on time. He does not look at any fixed point, but takes in many things at once. He pedals with a certain rhythm, without making brusque movements, as if each action arises from the previous one. He rides as if he does not need to intervene at all.

Anyone who has read *Zen and the Art of Archery*, in

which the arrow "fires itself" from the archer, would remark of such cyclists, "They let themselves ride." The action comes from the vital force that flows from the belly, not from the person who stretches the bowstring or turns the pedals (or from his ego); it comes from a supernatural force that manifests when the ego disappears. Cyclists who do not know of the existence of hara still draw their movements from that centre.

When you "unload" your torso onto the saddle, your legs are freed of their weight. They are raised, lowered and rotated rhythmically. More than putting pressure on the pedals, they "accompany" the perfect circle that the pedals describe through the air. More than resist the pressure that must be used to move the wheels, the pedals deliver themselves to the feet.

This way of spreading the driving force around the circle has something of the technique used by some racing cyclists. There is almost no difference between the moment in which they press down on the pedal and that in which the pedal lifts the foot. They push on the pedal in the same way during its entire revolution. When you watch them, you do not know whether they are using all their force, riding gently, or saving their strength. You don't see the least effort in their faces.

This form of "round" pedalling takes advantage of the rise of the foot and gains approximately 20 percent extra propulsion but is not a valid technique for urban cyclists because, in the middle of traffic, it is not convenient to use toe clips, straps, or anything that fixes the foot to the pedal. However, in the dynamics of round pedalling, there are two or three items that can be salvaged. The main one is that the force does not only come from the muscles of the legs but depends on how much you open your diaphragm: as it expands, your breathing reaches the abdomen. As we have already seen, a tense stomach and abdomen do not contribute to the flow of the vital force.

Cycling, along with jogging and swimming, comes at the top of the list of recommended aerobic activities. If you are going to make long journeys, your strategy must be to establish a "cadence of pedalling". In cycling jargon, cadence is the number of times that the pedal turns per minute. In beginners, there is a habitual tendency to maintain a low rate of cadence. Although it may seem paradoxical, if you make very little effort when pedalling it can cause injury to your knees. A common saying among long-distance cyclists is that your legs get tired at the same rate as your lungs. If your legs get tired before, this is a reminder that the cadence is too slow; if you tend to find yourself out of breath, it is too fast.

Although the cadence rate varies from one cyclist to another, a reasonable average is between 60 and 70 complete turns of the pedal per minute (decreasing when you climb a slope or increasing when there is even a minor downward slope). There are watches that indicate cadence, without the need to calculate it mentally.

Pedalling while concentrating on the here-and-now of the circular movement of the legs does not require you to fix your attention on the pedalling, and it stops the mind from going forward towards utilitarian thoughts such as, *If I pedal like this I will arrive faster and get less tired, etc.* All it means is that you are aware of what you are doing so that you can do it in the best way you can.

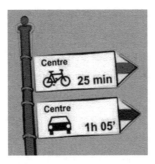

See and Anticipate

When you start riding a bike, and each time you go out on one, there is a natural tendency to look down at the area of ground beneath the front wheel and the handlebars and at the bit of road in front of you. The same look simultaneously captures what happens above and to the sides.

Once seated, the cyclist's head becomes one with the neck and trunk and almost does not move. You take in what is happening ahead only by moving the eyes and making use of your peripheral vision. You look at some point and see what is happening around you out of the corners of your eyes. This kind of "wide-angle" seeing that surrounds the central vision provides you with a context. Without looking at any point in particular you see everything in general. Each change, movement, or signal that appears in your field of vision is registered and decoded in terms of the progress that you are making (direction, speed, and so on). Long ago, Aristotle said that of all the senses, sight is the one that most allows us to acquire knowledge and discern "differences".

The eyes see and at the same time act as censors that record these small differences and draw conclusions. The more we know their meanings, the more we can "read" our unconscious in them. Gestures, lights, and the movements of other vehicles give us clues as to what other road users are going to do. If someone is standing on the curb at a corner, he may want to cross the road. If a car is going slowly, the driver might be looking for where to park; he could stop suddenly and only afterwards remember to indicate. If a car is stationary but has the front wheels twisted to one side, it probably wants to change lanes or overtake. If a bus cuts you off, it is possible that it is going to stop to drop off or pick up passengers, which will oblige you to brake or to pass it on the other side.

Much of the irritation that cyclists provoke in drivers is due to our unpredictability. In fairness, cars often drive in straight lines, follow lanes, refrain from weaving, and use their indicator lights... A bike offers you so much freedom that at times you believe you are the only person on the road and you can go where you want: down a corridor created by a row of parked cars; out in front of the cars waiting for a traffic light to change; the opposite direction down a one-way street; onto the pavement and along it at full speed...

The view from a bike is very different from the view from a car or from a bus. In those other forms of transport, windscreens and windows are television screens in which the scenes of the city parade, frame by frame. A bike does not have a roof, walls, or windows to separate the rider from the weather. With a circular view, going in all directions and also covering the ground and the sky, you have a feeling of being a part of what you see. It is a wonderful feeling, and at times it is highly enjoyable. However, if you are relaxed, this peripheral or "oceanic" way of seeing produces a mixture of hypnosis and disconnection, and this can put you at risk. It shifts you out of that state in which you are attentive to yourself and your surroundings, and in which, even though you are not aware of everything, you are alert to every sign. As in zazen and meditation, one way out of loss of concentration, or of numbness, is to focus on your breathing.

Breathe

"The energy of life in the universe that is contained in the air is transformed into human energy."
— *Taisen Deshimaru*

You cannot choose the air you breathe, but you can work with it until you find a rhythm in the inhalation and exhalation of it. Your awareness will integrate your breathing with the work of your muscles.

As my body breathes in and out automatically, I rarely remember that I am breathing or think about how I do it. I pedal, I get tired, my breaths become shorter, and I pant... I take in lungfuls of air and push them away again without paying much attention. In some streets, I notice the aroma of the trees; I inhale a little deeper, hold the air, and feel it. I may also be aware of breathing out, but in the next breath, or the one after that, I again become disconnected from my breathing.

If I become aware of the rhythm of my breathing, and of my diaphragm being released from tension, I am able to take breaths that reach farther down in the abdomen; the pressure of the rib cage transmits waves to the abdominal muscles and the muscles below. To draw in air from down there and send it out again requires me to take strength from the ocean of energy that is hara. All martial arts take advantage of the energy from this type of breathing, which emanates from the waist, kidneys, and hips. The key for the cyclist is to become gradually familiar with the route of the waves, and not block the flow through bad posture, or force it beyond its possibilities.

6

Look Out

The respect of motorists for cyclists stems not only from the fact that they see us but also how they see us. Wearing a helmet makes you conspicuous and is a warning, but it is only a passive safety measure in case anything happens to you. The active safety measure is to avoid a collision and/or fall in the first place — because the unthinkable always happens. You need to be aware of what could happen and anticipate the reaction of the other road user. If you cannot change the world, change the way you look at it.

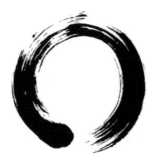

An Inner Code

If you can avoid it, it is not an accident.

The public enemies of the cyclist are not cars, buses, or missing manhole covers; the enemy is himself. His wavering attention, arrogance, recklessness, and—let's be honest—stupidity can turn against him. Such attitudes can lead to similar or greater problems than those caused by the drivers of motor vehicles, potholes in the road surface, or a lack of signs. Traffic regulations are quite ambiguous with regard to obligations. Hardly anyone obeys them in detail, and no one enforces them.

Many of the urban cyclist's forms of behaviour are "a-legal": neither legal or illegal, neither allowed nor prohibited. For example, can you ride down the middle lane of an avenue?

To take a one-way street in the wrong direction to save using two or three more streets, the cyclist risks getting trapped because there is not enough room. He may manage to get past an oncoming vehicle and be insulted by the driver, but he has actually broken the law. Nobody is going to fine him for this, but it is simply not the right thing to do. This lack of "righteousness" (what a word to apply to a cyclist!) contravenes a basic principle that goes even farther: that you must show respect if you want to be respected. Riding a bike well also has to do with the dharma, the search for your own nature.

We are living at a historic moment of cultural importance in which bike use is enjoying an exponential growth, thanks to a variety of factors. If cyclists do not learn to co-exist naturally with other road users, their behaviour will end up being regulated. In any regulation there is always a loss of freedom.

Urban cycling is now officially recognized; it has reached a stage of adulthood, and that means it has obligations. As soon as the cyclist realizes this and honours it as an inner law to abide by, he is able to change riding habits that seem to do no harm to anyone but create risk. Owning up to these patterns of behaviour, accepting the need to change them, and taking the decision to control them means to unlearn these habits, and this may take more time than learning to ride a bike.

A number of denials or justifications tempt the cyclist to violate the traffic regulations. You say to yourself: *I'll do it just this once; there's no one coming; I can't see anyone; I can get through that gap,* and so on. Sometimes, you don't even think about it and just do it directly. The fact that most times it turns out alright and nothing happens does not eliminate the possibility that one day it may go wrong. This anarchic nature needs to be channelled.

You do not go through a red light, even if no one is coming from the side road. You do not go in the wrong direction down a street. You do not drive on motorways or across bridges where human-powered vehicles are prohibited. You do not ride on pavements. You do not carry another adult on the back, not even on the luggage rack, much less on the handlebars, and you don't carry bags hanging off the handlebars, either. You do not zig-zag. You don't do wheelies. You do not use your mobile phone... Any of these and other small acts, even if they appear insignificant, may complicate life more than you can imagine.

You do not *not* do these things solely because of the possible consequences; you refrain from them because they hurt the spirit of the cyclist—when you deviate from proper conduct, you produce a break inside yourself, even if you don't have an accident. To do these things impedes cycling from becoming an activity that encourages harmony, both inside the cyclist and with all those around him. For pedestrians, drivers, and passengers looking out of the window of a bus, the sight of a cyclist can create a resonance of spirit. Another proof of this: when you see someone bend down to pick up the droppings left by his dog on the pavement and dispose of them in a plastic bag, doesn't it make you think about what is right and wrong?

Riding a bike makes people friendlier and forces them to be responsible. By complying with the rules of travelling in the city, and with the dictates of common sense, each of us aligns himself with the higher order and resets the pattern of energy. In some way, it also protects us. A motorist that sees a cyclist being careful with his own space and the public space may be inspired by such an attitude to imitate it. At least, he will look at cyclists in another way.

"The eye has a thousand eyes,
like the Bodhisattva of Compassion.
Each one is a hand looking for a cushion in the darkness."
—*George Leonard*

7

Keep It Impeccable

Any noise, loose part, uneven wear, lack of oil, or breakage
means that something is not working as it should.
The cyclist develops a sensitivity to such warnings.
It is not necessary to be an expert to apply preventive
logic. To observe the components —
noting them one by one and allowing them to show us
how they work — leads to an understanding
of what may be wrong with them.

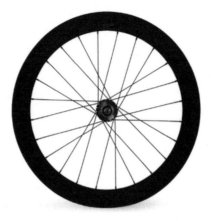

> *"What is Zen?" asks a young man.*
> *"Have you had your tea?" answers the master.*
> *"Yes."*
> *"And did you wash up the cup?"*
> *"Yes."*
> *"Well, that is Zen."*
> —*Story narrated by Thomas Merton*

Zen has an expression that integrates the presence of body, mind, and attitude in the immediate present. Where we are when we do something, where the mind is, and what the body is doing. It literally and specifically means to be attentive to the action—to keep the mind from going somewhere else other than the present moment and the body from doing something other than what is most appropriate. If I am sawing a piece of wood, it is best to keep my mind's eye on the cut I am making; if I polish it afterwards, to keep my mind on the polishing. In preparing my piece of wood, I should aim to remove my internal view from the end result, from what I will achieve through my work, and focus instead on each stage of the process as closely as possible. Observation of action, concentration on the doing rather than the goal: this is the meaning of *samu*.

Once something is achieved it is no longer anything, say Zen masters. It was.

Before and After

Some time ago, I was at a spiritual retreat centre. They were building new dormitories, and I was assigned to carpentry work, specifically to make the windows. Every day, we had to meditate with the tools for 15 minutes before starting our tasks and stop work half an hour before the scheduled time to do the same. Wherever we were, we stopped and took that time to clean our tools, one by one, while we reflected in silence on the experience. The objective was to remove any vestige of sawdust and wipe an oily rag over any metal surface. We had to sharpen the chisels. We had to put the drill bits back in their cases, arranged in order from the largest to the smallest. Similarly, we had to sort the screws, nuts, and bolts by their sizes. We had to clean the teeth of the saw. Then we had to store each tool in the same place from which we had taken it. Finally, we dusted the work surfaces and swept the floor of the workshop. The next time our group or any other came in they would find everything as if nobody had ever been in here. Once the workshops had been tidied, we went around and thanked the tools for the tasks they had facilitated.

If someone from outside had seen all this they may have said that we were being a little exaggerated. Those of us who were there knew—as anyone who has ever spent time in a Zen community knows—that loving care of the tools, almost as if they were human, had the same value as any other spiritual practice undertaken at that centre. There was not an "us" on one side and tools on another. The ritual was to remind us that we are both instruments of a same sole, unifying energy.

To return to the tools in the evening or the next day, the feeling that they produced in our hands said it all. To be reunited with them immediately created an internal sense of alignment with them, and this was the aim of the centre. It was the same experience for those who worked in the kitchen, in the garden, on the looms, building walls, or in the offices: they all took time to begin and end their work. If any novice like me did not understand on arrival, by the next day he understood.

Taking Care of It Is Taking Care of Myself

The actress Michele Pfeiffer confessed several times that she relaxed by taking her bicycle to pieces and reassembling it. Hemingway said something about writing that also applies to cyclists and bicycles: "You are the one who really knows what is not working."

Bicycle maintenance is also a metaphor for what we do with ourselves. Often the first thing you want to do when you return from a trip is open the fridge, leaving the bike in the state that it arrived in, leaning against a wall, forgotten. The next day, you pick it up, turn it around, and go out again.

I am not saying that you should thank it for the services provided on each journey—although why not?—or service it daily. However, to become aware of its "life" and of the effects that use has on its parts can give you guidance on what works in a particular way and not in another. A connection is created that transcends that of user-machine. By taking care of it, you take care of yourself. I take care of "us" (it and me) and thus I ride aligned.

It follows that to clean my bike is to clean my mind. When I align or tune it, I align myself. To give it time when I am not riding it is a way to be with—and to know about—myself. I give myself peace of mind, because what happens outside happens inside.

While he cycles, the cyclist feels the rubbing of the tyre on the road surface, the clicking of chain links as they pass from one sprocket to another, and the functioning of various other components. He does not see; he feels or hears. His connection or perception of the operation of his vehicle allows him to detect any malfunction, even intuitively, sometimes before it occurs. If the wheel is not correctly balanced and centred between the brake blocks; if the pressure has dropped in one of the inner tubes; if there is an irregularity or stiffness in the chain; if the handlebar is loose—the body is "alerted" to the problem. In the same natural way in which the cyclist keeps his balance or moves between other vehicles, something automatic operates within him related to the care of the machine. Each cyclist knows the strengths and weaknesses of his own bike, its structural flaws and idiosyncrasies. The more you use your bike, the more receptive you become to its symptoms.

You don't notice a perfectly adjusted bicycle. It lets you pedal it; it gives you a smooth ride; it is strong and silent (no part complains); and it integrates your movements, as if it was an extension of your anatomy. It puts up almost no resistance: all parts instantly interpret your signals, whether you want to go forwards, brake, or change gear.

It is essential to make regular adjustments to avoid a progressive deterioration caused by the lack of lubrication or the play of some loose component. Each time you return home, you can at least give it a quick check. It is not always possible to get down on your knees to adjust or repair something that has come loose or broken with use, but it is possible to become aware of such things, so that they do not take you by surprise the next time you want to ride it. The ritual of checking creates a meditation space between the recent riding of the bicycle and the riding to come. If the bike is part of you, this moment gives its use another meaning.

When you approach your bike with affection and start to lose your fear of its mechanics, you realize that everything has its logic and that some parts can be disassembled without fear. Once you have successfully carried out some task of adjustment or repair you will be inspired to go farther. Initial steps include straightening the brake pads, oiling the chain, tightening any nut or a screw that moves, and checking the position of the handlebars. Little by little, as you understand the logic of assembly and operation, you will feel more confident about tackling other parts.

There are annual or biannual servicing routines that are best left to someone skilled. However, many small tasks of weekly or monthly maintenance require a minimum of specific knowledge and only a certain amount of patience—that never goes amiss—and two or three tools.

The Logic of Inference

A craftsman does not always follow a single line of instructions, because decisions are required as the work progresses. The nature of the material in his hands determines his thoughts and movements. Robert Pirsig says this in *Zen and the Art of Motorcycle Maintenance*. A few lines farther down, he explains that, at the conclusion of the work, the mind rests in a different way if the work has been mechanical.

You achieve peace of mind when you have managed to resolve the issues that worry you. This means: to be willing to repair things; to be detached; and to have the clarity of mind necessary to confront any issues or problems that may be pending or unresolved.

To ride in peace, because all the parts are working well, is a reasonable idea for a speculative mind accustomed to setting objectives. According to Zen, if you are not at peace when you go out on a bike ride, or while you are working on maintenance, it is very likely that you give your personal problems to your bike.

In other words, the bicycle can be perfect, but if you find something that disturbs you about it or your own reality, it will not work flawlessly until your mind is serene.

The attitude of a Zen practitioner is like that of a true specialist or a craftsman, or of anyone who invest themselves to what they do without a full set of instructions: it is let each step tell you what to do next. This prevents technical know-how from slowing the intuition down.

The logic of Zen breaks the logic of cause and consequence on which inference is based. To infer is to deduce one thing from another by what emerges from it, through reasoning. Riding a bike is concrete proof that this system works: it does not follow any set of written instructions. As you proceed, absorbed and attentive to what you are doing, even if you are not doing it deliberately, you are making an infinite number of decisions by inference every second.

That half hour that we used to set aside in the community to put the tools back in their original state after we had used them was indeed an external form of letting go of the task performed; it was a meditation in action that allowed the mind to settle. The minutes before and after a bike ride seem to have the same sense as the ride itself, but they are not the same; they are parts of a harmonious whole. To leave all the parts clean, well organized, and ready for when you need to use them again, without the "baggage" of previous use, makes for an eloquent relationship with the inner self. I am also that set of parts.

"THE PERSON WHO CLEANS IS NOT HERE.
THE PEOPLE WHO ARE HERE DO NOT CLEAN.
THEREFORE, PLEASE LEAVE EVERYTHING
AS CLEAN AS IT WAS."
—*Sign in a classroom-workshop*

Epilogue 1

My Seven Bikes

Whenever I arrive in a city, my priority is to get a bike.
Then I feel like a local.

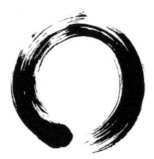

*"Your first bicycle ride contains all the trips
that you are going to make in your life. [...]
To get on a bike for the first time was an act of initiation.
It meant that you had to leave the family
to lose yourself on an unknown route."*
—Manuel Vicent

When I was three years old, my parents gave me my first bike: a 16" Broadway "with little wheels", as we called stabilizers then. In 1982, when I was just over 38, I began to use a 28" Raleigh almost every day, and I discovered that the bicycle is much more than a means of transport, recreation, sport, or other form of exercise. Unintentionally, every time I get my bike out to go to the centre or to go for a ride ("distances that are no deterrent to pedalling", as Eduardo Galeano puts it), I have perceptions that in general I am not aware of, both about what I see, and about the phenomenon of cycling.

The city is the same, and at the same time seems to me to be different. It activates in me a primal energy, something very close to happiness. Between the Broadway and the Raleigh, I had several bicycles: seven in total.

When the stabilizers were removed from that first bike, riding became like a game, the same as running after a ball, or hitting it with a bat. I was keen to know how little I could move my legs and still keep moving; at what speed I would begin to get scared; which of the boys of my street would be first to the corner or take less time to go around the block; which of us could go the longest time without using hands; which of us was able to stand with one foot on the saddle and lift the other; who could zigzag between tin cans, placed increasingly closer to each other, without falling off.

When I was alone, I set myself another dare: how far could I go? (always beyond the limits set by my parents). After that, the bike became connected with growing up: I insisted on having a 24", like the bikes my brothers would not lend me. When my parents bought them an adult bike, an Italian Bianchi racer, the only one in the neighbourhood, they gave me the 24". To get on it, I had to tilt it 45 degrees to have my feet on the ground. When I rode it through the streets of Castelar, the town where we lived, I felt grown up. However, it never became mine.

My mother used her own bike—a gold-coloured Phillips—twice a week to go to a market located on the other side of the train tracks. She would return with the baskets full and with two huge bags hanging from the handlebars. Until shortly before her death, her face would look younger when she remembered those moments. She had learned to ride when she was an adult, after we were born. The first or the second time that she got on the golden bike, a present from my father, she fell off on to a pile of dung newly dropped by the horse that was pulling the baker's cart. Every time she told the story she would exclaim, "It was steaming!"

To go with my mother's bike, my father bought a metallic blue bike for weekends, but it didn't last very long. On the day that he brought it home, he didn't close the gate properly and someone took it. He got so angry that he said he would never get another one or get on one. After the theft, he never went out with us, not even on my elder brother's bike, nor that of my mother. Two attitudes to life.

While we lived in that town, my brothers and I used to use the bikes for any excuse, even to ride to the corner. We also went by bike to any friend's house—we took them just to have them available. It looked more important if we arrived pedalling rather than on foot, even if the bike was left lying on the ground, forgotten, for the rest of the afternoon.

When we moved to the centre of the city, we only took the Bianchi with us. For a few months, it stayed in the basement of the building, behind a Provençal bookcase. Until one Saturday, when I got it out and took it to have the wheels pumped up and went to explore Costanera Avenue. Everyone at home said, it is dangerous for a 12-year-old boy to be riding among the cars... but it was already too late, because I had claimed the bike for myself.

The Bianchi had no inner tubes or tyres, only yellow-and-black tubes that always had to be inflated to the maximum pressure. A cigarette butt on the road made them jump, to say nothing of a stone, or a ride across the tram tracks. The cobbled streets were impossible.

My new school friends and my friends at the club thought it was very provincial for me to arrive and leave on a bicycle.

What teenage boy in those days didn't wish for the chance to carry the girl of his dreams sitting on the handlebars, looking towards him, holding onto him with her hands around his neck? Many people have seen it in films; others imagine it as something natural. To those of us who considered the bike to be part of ourselves, it was a metaphor for the happiness promised by a relationship.

The desire to ride a bike lessened when I started to drive my father's car. Until I got my first Citroen 2CV, when I was 25, I had one of the first Honda 50 motorcycles in the country and my brothers had a Siambretta. In the meantime, without our consent and without our knowing, our parents gave the Bianchi to the son of the doorman.

I forgot how much I liked to ride a bike until one of those twists of fate in life brought it back to me. I was nearly 30 and working in an advertising agency in Paris. I realized that the Metro took away the opportunity to see—and live in—the city. I was discussing this with the owner of the apartment that I was renting, when he offered me a bicycle that he no longer used; if I looked after it (and carried it up and down three flights of stairs), I could use it whenever I want. He explained, however, "It is still mine." It was a classic 28" Peugeot, and very smooth to ride. I mention the brand because of the significance it had for me, a South American, to discover that the factory that made the cars after which we all hankered also made such "lesser" vehicles. I didn't know then how important they had been before, during and after the Second World War. When I climbed the hills of Sacré-Coeur and St-Cloud riding "our" Peugeot, I had my own experience of the existential cycling fervour of Henry Miller in his Parisian period.

During the oil crisis of 1973, the Arab countries demonstrated the power they had by turning off the tap and shaking the prosperity of Europe. In Paris, young people, students, men in suits, and working women got around on mopeds. The Mobilette and the Solex were part of everyday life.

In the streets, they left me behind. They cost very little, used almost no fuel, and could be parked anywhere. However, out of a mixture of pride and loyalty, I stuck to that outdated machine that you have to pedal.

That same year, the agency designed a campaign to attract subscriptions for *Le Sauvage*, a monthly magazine dedicated to ecology—a word that still sounded mysterious—launched by *Le Nouvel Observateur*, the weekly periodical of the non-radical left. I suggested we use the silhouette of a bicycle as a symbol. At the meeting in which we presented our sketches to the publishers and advertisers, they responded that they were looking for something else. Their arguments were: bicycles belong to the past; we associate them with austerity; we want something more alive. Finally, they opted for the raised arm of someone calling for help from the middle of a lake full of bottles and plastic waste.

Shortly afterwards, life took me to London. It took me 20 minutes to get from the Underground station to work. My weekly ticket cost the equivalent of half a day's pay. While I was deciding whether or not to buy a bike, I found one that was almost wrecked in a container. I heaved it over my shoulder, took it to pieces completely, placed all of the parts in a jar of petrol to soak, and took the whole thing to the neighbourhood bike shop. Fifteen days later, for a charge that today I remember as a pittance, they gave me back a beautiful bike, ready to ride, painted blue and white.

"Very *Argie*," they announced. "You're right," I said, "it is very Argentinian." Now I needed to buy a raincoat especially for cyclists. I am not the only crazy person. Many English people I knew in those years were stubborn enough to cycle in the rain. Five years later, a few days before going back to my own country, I sold my bike to a Peruvian boy who had just arrived. I didn't want to think about how much I would miss it.

I bought my fifth bike from Pedrinho, a bicycle man in Búzios (a fishing town north of Rio de Janeiro), where I spent almost three years. Pedrinho lived in a shack in Vila Caranga, amidst the debris of bikes left behind by tourists that couldn't be fixed any more. Everyone considered him to be the village idiot. I chose a bike that would work on any terrain, that would especially stand up to the beach and not be too affected by rust. It was so basic that I could leave it anywhere without worrying about it being stolen. No one would want to even borrow it. It was my most faithful companion at that time.

My mother (68 years old at the time) decided to spend some time with me. The first thing we did was visit Pedrinho. While we climbed the hill behind his hut-workshop to watch one of the most beautiful sun-sets in the world, he readied a small-wheeled bicycle that was very similar to today's folding models. The next day, coming back from the beach, I wanted my mother to try it out and get to know Praia dos Osos.

"Do you dare to go up to the headland and return through Tartaruga?" I asked her.

"I haven't been on a bike for a quarter of a century," she replied.

When I saw her set off pedalling, it looked as if she had never got off. Suddenly, going down a dip, her bike started to pick up speed. I started racing towards her, but I estimated that I would not be able to reach her before she lost control. Even if I could catch up with her, what would I do? I only managed to shout: "Brake, Mum, brake, Muuum...!" Pedrinho must have used a few pieces of rubber cut up in any old way as brake pads.

I blamed myself for my irresponsibility in having exposed her to this danger. I did not want to think what was going to happen in the next few seconds. I watched as she gripped the frame with her legs and kept herself straight until the end of the descent. Then she let the speed reduce by itself.

We stopped to rest. I checked that her brakes were in perfect working condition.

"Why didn't you apply them?" I chided her.

"What did you want me to do?" she answered. "Lock them and kill myself?"

A couple of months afterwards, before returning to Argentina, she said, "Shall we take them home with us?" I don't know why I refused.

Back in Buenos Aires, I planned outings as if I still had a bike. I rented an office six streets from where I lived, and I moved around within a radius of 4,000–5,000 metres (2.5–3 miles). It was 1982, and very few people were cycling then.

Chia would be the only mother with a bike, waiting for school to let out. She had a large and wide one, with two seats: one hanging from the handlebars backwards, the other bolted to the rear luggage rack. "Shall we go and see what colour the lake is today?" she would say to the children, as she put them on the bike. Almost every day, Jazmín (5) and Fede (4) earned a ride around the Palermo woods before going home.

Mountain bikes had not yet arrived in the country; replicas of traditional European bikes are still manufactured but in reduced numbers, with a crossbar for men and without a crossbar for women, so they don't need to lift a leg to climb on. By coincidence, someone, the ex-husband of a girl I know in a meditation group, had imported a consignment of Raleigh bikes—the classic black model with a Brooks leather saddle—and he wanted to promote them. I went to see him, we did a deal, and I returned riding. It was a sign.

I used it. I would look at it leaning against the bookcase in my apartment or behind my desk, and even when I just thought about it, the feeling was the same: I had been reunited with that part of me that, even without being able to define happiness, had been happy many times.

I watched them pass me, and I would say to myself, *Mountain bikes are not for me*. That is, until one Sunday in 1990, when I tried one in the country house of some friends of mine. That same week I bought a similar model, a Specialized Zenith with Shimano gears. My thumbs immediately imprinted their function on my neural pathways. I gave the black Raleigh—immortalized on the cover of the first issue of *Uno Mismo* magazine, and every day used to make a hundred trips to the editorial office—to Federico, who had got tired of his BMX, a red Fiorenza, and already had long enough legs for an adult bike.

That mountain bike survived everything. An accident in which Clara, my youngest daughter, then three years old, was sitting on the crossbar, when she slid her toes between the spokes of the front wheel, and we both went flying over the handlebars. Consequence: plaster and scars. It survived a Honda Express that my niece Violet lent me, and it survived a green and powerful Vespa 250—a childhood dream of mine.

It even survived a 48cc Chinese engine, which I attached to the frame and removed soon after because it had made it something other than a bicycle. It survived a time when I forgot it in the doorway of a bar. And the temptation to change it... I love it as a former companion in arms.

As I write this book, it never ceases to amaze me the variety of models that I see on the streets of Buenos Aires and the designs of electric bikes that have been created by the major car brands. As a whim of maturity, I got it into my head to go back to riding a classic English. Those that I could find on the Internet in Argentina and Uruguay were no longer in their original state. In addition, their owners wanted to sell them as antiques. One morning, I remembered that Ino Iaccarino, one of the editors of *Uno Mismo*, had bought a bike similar to mine, when we did the first few editions of the magazine. I called to ask if he still had it. His answer gave me goosebumps, "It is waiting for you." An '83 Roadmaster—what a name—dark green, Brooks saddle, Sturmey Archer gears, and dynamo in the rear axle... It even had the original transfers. I did not even need to oil it to make it go.

"We always go back to the same places," said Jazmín, who had just bought a bike with a seat behind. Manu (then two), my first grandson, rides to and from kindergarten in the same manner his mother once rode to school, when I met her. When I see Clara pull out her blue-and-white Canaglia to go to work, or when I receive photos of Brian and Kirsten riding together in Denmark or through Central Park in New York, I feel something similar, for which I have no words...

Nothing else. Only this. To ride and to see other people riding bikes awakens in me this kind of joy.

Epilogue 2

A Secular Zen

*Is it possible to consider yourself a Zen practitioner
without always following a master,
or undertaking disciplined practice within a congregation?
Do you need to be ordained?
What determines whether or not you are Zen?*

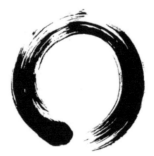

"The fruits ripen by themselves."
—Bodhidharma

When I was 16, I read Eugen Herrigel's *Zen and the Art of Archery*, and I was hit by a realization: the student must stand on the shoulders of the teacher. If necessary, he must kill him.

I hear the same message shouted by the beatnik poet Allen Ginsberg: Don't follow anyone. Krishnamurti, another person that I read at that time, is more categorical: Be your own master.

Right! So, everything I have been told may or may not be true; the only thing that can stay with me is what comes from me. It comes from listening to what I say to myself, and from the truthfulness with which I answer myself.

The role of the master (*roshi*), as I understand it, is to help me tune into that little voice inside; my own voice, before the arrival of words; the voice that has been silenced by parents, teachers, culture, membership groups... or by my fears.

Beyond the truth that I may attribute to these messages, I still find it hard to understand that Buddhism and Zen are something that goes from the inside to the outside.

All things considered, from then on, even without being able to explain it much, I feel part of that family.

I have only been into Zen meditation halls (*dojos*) four or five times. I never felt comfortable wearing the black tunic or entering from the left. Only on a few occasions have I met a master. I have never undertaken retreats in monasteries or participated in any ceremony. Sometimes, I have meditated in groups; other times, in private; but I cannot say I have a diploma in meditation.

I have a lot of respect for anyone who finds, or makes, a space for himself within such a framework. More than their persistence, I appreciate the friendliness with which they act, and I share their vows: to reconnect with my own Buddhahood; refrain from lying, stealing, killing; acknowledge the suffering of others as my own... Over the years, these ideals have come to seem natural to me. As a commitment to myself.

My relationship with Zen seems to go by other routes.

I am relieved that Zen does not speak of God, but of non-duality. Things and beings—all of them have interdependent existences. Everything is connected and is part of a whole. The one, unique thing. Limits and dualistic thinking are products of the mind.

Zen does not offer divinities that you can worship. Nor is there a reward in the hereafter. Although Zen speaks of attaining *satori*, it does not say you have to look to it as a goal. It speaks of awakening before each experience. Practice and enlightenment are not different things.

It does not provide answers; it makes each of us seek his own, even without the intention of finding them. You seek for the sake of seeking, without clinging to certainties.

There is no series of steps or levels to be accomplished. Much of the learning consists of unlearning: dismantling models for the understanding of reality that have taken root as preconceptions within our thoughts; letting go of ideas that we consider definitive; allowing discoveries to surprise our passions; not making decisions based simply on impressions or emotions...

Personally, I am attracted by Zen's non-moralistic, non-devotional, and non-proselytizing character. No monk or Zen practitioner I have ever met has done anything to convince me in the least. His truth includes accepting all the truths that other people may have. My truth is to remember this.

When someone puts his hands together and bows his head (*gassho*) to someone, or before the figure of Buddha, he owns his own Buddha nature and that of being in front of him: the Buddha salutes the Buddha.

In some schools, Zen is *zazen*: the discipline of sitting cross-legged in contemplation with your eyes closed and, through the correct posture and breathing, entering into a state of emptiness or nothingness. But all practitioners consider that zazen continues, or is just beginning, when you get up from your cushion.

Zazen is an attitude present in all the activities of life. In each place, in every moment. Zen is always there, whatever you do. Everything can be a form of Zen, whatever you want to call it—but better not to give it a name at all.

In the Vimalakirti Sutra, there is an eloquent anecdote. Several practitioners meet to talk about emptiness. After each one gives his interpretation, the Bodhisattva Manjushri, personification of the Supreme Wisdom, says that as soon as you speak, you are making a mistake. A lay practitioner present among them watches in silence—in "a deafening silence", says the Sutra. Manjushri approves. His understanding exceeds that of all the others.

Certainly, for zazen to be something more than a discreet form of meditation—and in the first stage, it teaches you to abandon the body and the mind—it is essential that someone instructs you in the correct position and attitude. A good friend with experience, as many teachers are considered to be.

A partner on the journey, without other objectives, connotations or masks.

I mentioned the hand of the adult who holds the seat of the child who wants to learn to ride a bike.

The teachings do not constitute an identity of belonging. Nobody is a true Zen practitioner just because he is part of a group or Zen community; nor because he shares a feeling or a common belief with others. It is a solitary practice, which can be done with others, but as a "community of loners" (Giuseppe *Jiso* Forzani).

Neither does Zen obey a hierarchical institution, nor promote power structures. An ordained monk, a practitioner, and an independent (I am reluctant to say secular, because I do not consider Zen to be a religion) are equal because they are all engaged on the same search: for their own nature.

Since the time of the Buddha, countless people have taken on his teachings and practised his precepts—without the need to follow any master, without having been ordained, and without belonging to any congregation. Without even calling what they do Zen.

They do not question whether they are or are not Zen. They experience it with total freedom, without expecting anything in return, and without being answerable to anyone but themselves.

At times—as cyclists know well—you can get to the same destination by two parallel paths. There can be Zen in releasing a bow string, blowing a bamboo flute, or serving a cup of tea.

Theoretically, a cyclist is not a Zen practitioner, but what he does can be considered Zen. Who is he, but what he does?

"That" which is experienced on each ride.

There is not "one" single Buddhism, one Zen, one explanation. There are as many as there are personal experiences. Out of all that you hear about it or that you read (including in this book), Zen is what resonates with you. If the little voice tells you not to follow such and such a bicycle lane or to turn in a particular place, there may be a reason.

Detours are also part of the road.

The great journey is nothing else but recovering the original mind.

Bibliography

Al Chung-Liang Huang. *Embrace Tiger, Return to Mountain: The Essence of T'ai Chi*. Moab, Utah: Real People Press, 1973.

Augé, Marc. *Éloge de la bicyclette*. Paris: Payot et Rivages, 2008.

Baigorria, Osvaldo. *Buda y las religiones sin Dios*. Buenos Aires-Madrid: Campo de Ideas, 2002.

Byrne, David. *Bicycle Diaries*. New York: Viking Penguin, 2009.

Caddy, Eileen. *God Spoke to Me*. Forres: Findhorn Press, 1971.

Caddy, Eileen & D. E. Platts (ed.). *Opening Doors Within*. Forres: Findhorn Press, 1986.

Coomaraswamy, Ananda K. *The Symbolism of Archery*. Michigan: Ars Islamica, 1943.

Dürckheim, K.G. *Hara, the Vital Centre of Man*. London: Allen & Unwin, 1962.

Glassman, B. & Fields, R. *Instructions to the Cook: A Zen Master's Lesson in Living a Life That Matters*. New York: Bell Tower, 1996.

Herrigel, Eugen. *Zen and the Art of Archery* (Introduction by D.T. Suzuki). New York: Pantheon, 1953.

Honoré, Carl. *In Praise of Slowness: Challenging the Cult of Speed*. New York: HarperCollins, 2004.

McCluggage, Denise. *The Centered Skier*. Vermont: Crossroads, 1977.

Pirsig, R. *Zen and the Art of Motorcycle Maintenance*. New York: William Morrow, 1974.

Nachmanovitch, Stephen. *Free Play. Improvisation in Life and Art*. New York: Tarcher/Putnam, 1990.

Reps, Paul (compiler). *Zen Flesh, Zen Bones*. Boston, Massachusetts: Tuttle, 1957.

Suzuki, D. T. *The Zen Doctrine of No Mind and Essays in Zen Buddhism*. New York: Rider, 1969.

Suzuki, Shunryu. *Zen Mind, Beginner's Mind*. Boulder, Colorado: Weatherhill/Shambhala, 1970.

Thich Nhat Hanh. *Present Moment, Wonderful Moment*. Escondido, California: Unified Buddhist Church, 1990.

Villalba, Dokusho. *¿Qué es el Zen? Introducción práctica al budismo Zen*. Madrid: Miraguano Ediciones, 1984.

Watts, Allan. *This Is It and Other Essays on Zen and Spiritual Experience*. New York: Vintage, 1960.

Acknowledgements

My mother used to come back from the market loaded with bags. Chia went to yoga classes by bicycle. My daughter Clara seems to have inherited my passion for the bike. Román Ripoll told me about "doing without doing";

Ricardo Benadón about the man-vehicle connection. Gerardo Abboud was always ready to clarify any doubts about Buddhism. Pancho Hunneus, Gustavo Ressia, and Agustin Paniker published books that opened my mind. César Civita entrusted me with the *abracadabra* of publishers: put a bicycle in the first edition of any new periodical. Gustavo Borenstein, Alberto and Ino Iaccarino were infected by my enthusiasm and created the necessary infrastructure so that the magazine *Uno Mismo* would come out every month. Héctor Pivernus and Cristina Grigna granted me the honour of making a special edition of *Zen and the Art of Archery* by Eugen Herrigel. Thich Nhat Hanh authorized me to translate his books *Present Moment, Wonderful Moment* and *The Sun My Heart*. Ricardo Parada, went from "distrust" to trust to be proved correct. Jorge Alberto explained to me how movement arises from imbalance and other physical laws that we use without knowing about them. Juan Manuel de los Reyes repaired my shattered elbow. Jorge (Ryúnan) Bustamante taught me that the meaning of the practice is beyond any theoretical elaboration. Edgardo Werbin Brener reinterpreted many of my experiences through Zen. Sebastian Donadío generously shared his technical expertise with me and Bob Curto his Zen erudition. Emilio Fernandez Cicco stripped my text of all artifice, until the book found itself. My brothers Osvaldo and Eduardo, and my dear family, were always by my side, as true travelling companions. Without them, this book would not be what it is...

About the Author

Juan Carlos Kreimer (bicizenjck@gmail.com) was born in Buenos Aires in 1944. He is a cultural journalist, writer, and editor. His books about rock music—*Beatles & Co* (1968), *¡Agarrate!* (1970), and *Punk: La Muerte Joven* (1978)—were the first on the subject to be published in Spanish. In 1982, he founded, and directed for 12 years, the magazine *Uno Mismo*. He is also the author of *¿Cómo Lo Escribo?* (1981), *Contracultura Para Principiantes, El Varón Sagrado, Rehacerse Hombres*, and three novels: *Todos lo Sabíamos, El Río y el Mar*, and *¿Quién Lo Hará Posible?*

Since 1995, he has been the editor of the Spanish version of the *For Beginners* series and of De La Flor's graphic novels. He has adapted two novels—*Los dueños de la tierra* by David Viñas and *The Stranger* by Albert Camus—as graphic novels. Two of his previous books have appeared in English: *Krishnamurti for Beginners* (Writers and Readers Publishing Inc., London, 1998) and *Counterculture for Beginners* (Zidane Press, London, 2017). He teaches a course on "Self-Discovery Through Writing" at the Colombia Foundation.

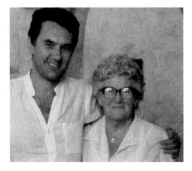

The author with Eileen Caddy, co-founder of the Findhorn Foundation